THE SMART GUIDE TO

Fighting Infections

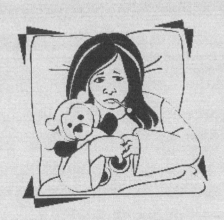

BY ANNE MACZULAK

The Smart Guide To Fighting Infections

Published by

Smart Guide Publications, Inc.
2517 Deer Chase Drive
Norman, OK 73071
www.smartguidepublications.com

For information, address: Smart Guide Publications, Inc. 2517 Deer Creek Drive, Norman, OK 73071

SMART GUIDE and Design are registered trademarks licensed to Smart Guide Publications, Inc.

International Standard Book Number: 978-1-937636-18-0

Library of Congress Catalog Card Number:
11 12 13 14 15   10 9 8 7 6 5 4 3 2 1

Printed in the United States of America

Cover design: Lorna Llewellyn
Copy Editor: Ruth Strother
Back cover design: Joel Friedlander, Eric Gelb, Deon Seifert
Back cover copy: Eric Gelb, Deon Seifert
Illustrations: James Balkovek
Production: Zoë Lonergan
Indexer: Cory Emberson
V.P./Business Manager: Cathy Barker

ACKNOWLEDGMENTS

I would like to thank the microbiologists that I have worked with and learned from during my years in the laboratory. Primary among these scientists are Charles Gerba, Philip Tierno, Rick Danielson, Mark Sobsey, Robin Dias, Carlos Enriquez, Wanda Manhanke, Carole Parnes, Judy Ikawa, and Allan Branch.

My appreciation also goes to Smart Guide's Frank Jerome and my agent Jodie Rhodes for developing the idea for this book and the superb editorial help of Ruth Strother, who did an extraordinary job editing this book. I also thank illustrator James Balkovek, who did a wonderful job illustrating the book.

Last but not least, I owe special gratitude to my writers group. We have supported and encouraged each other for many years. My writing career would not have begun without the inspiration I received from Sheldon Siegel, Priscilla Royal, Bonnie DeClark, Meg Stiefvater, and Janet Wallace.

TABLE OF CONTENTS

INTRODUCTION

Fighting Infection

This Book

What do we mean when we say we are going to fight infection? It could mean driving from the body an illness that has taken hold of you and making you feel miserable. You know something is wrong by your urge to sneeze or cough, headache and fatigue that make the simplest tasks a challenge, and by an ominous rumbling in the bowels. You would certainly do all in your power to get rid of such a feeling.

While you may resort to chicken soup and a good night's sleep, your body is waging furious warfare against the "bug" you have caught. This book gives you tips on bolstering your body's natural defenses against mild and more serious infections.

A second important piece to fighting infection exists, however, and it involves steps everyone should take to prevent germs from getting into the body in the first place. These prevention steps are more effective in maintaining good health than anything else you can do.

This *Smart Guide to Fighting Infections* tells you how to make a two-pronged attack against germs. First, it covers the actions you can take to keep germs from getting near you. But some germs will get through from time to time; it's inevitable. Therefore, this book also gives you information on what to do to help your body eliminate infection. You can make choices that help your body annihilate a germ as quickly as possible.

The 24 chapters in this book guide you through the basics of infection, including the microbes that cause infections and the diseases that sometimes develop from mild, localized infections. After learning the basics of the infection process and microbes, you will learn about toxins, which are poisons that microbes make. You will become familiar with the ways microbes get into your body and how they leave. You will also meet the microbes that live in harmony with you for most of your life but can betray you and cause illness if given the right opportunity.

This *Smart Guide* presents the big picture of epidemiology, or how scientists monitor the movement of disease through our population. The book gives you vital details on germ transmission. You cannot stop germs from reaching you if you don't know how they're transmitted from person to person!

Not to be forgotten are the food-borne and waterborne illnesses to which sooner or later we all fall victim. Some of these infections are merely pesky inconveniences; others are serious life-threatening events. In fact, that might be said for all infections. Some are mild;

some are serious. This book will guide you through the features of microbes that make them either dangerous foes or minor pests. The book also explains how your health has a direct influence on whether those germs cause mild illness or much more serious disease.

You will learn the nuts and bolts of your immune system, which is the silent process within your body that shields you from most infections. This book additionally gives you the basics of vaccines, hospital infections, new infections emerging today, and the illnesses we catch from animals.

Included in each chapter are sidebars that focus on five different aspects of microbiology. Certain sidebars give you added information on Microbe Basics. Others focus on Infections in History, in which events from past outbreaks affect you today, even though they happened a generation ago or longer. A sidebar called At the Doctor's Office helps you become better informed about infection diagnosis and treatment. Finally, sidebars that focus on Infections and Disease and Infection Vocabulary make this book a resource on the germs you're likely to meet someday.

Now, begin your tour of your body's infection-fighting tools, the germs you should know, and the places where we get infections.

PART ONE

Microbes and Infection

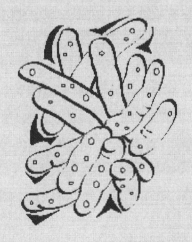

CHAPTER 1

What Is Infection?

In This Chapter

➤ Defining infection and distinguishing it from disease

➤ The main microbes that cause infection

➤ Basic information about infection and disease

➤ Examples of the most prevalent infectious diseases

➤ Defining normal flora, opportunistic pathogens, and how they relate

---

In this chapter, you'll learn what an infection is. Infection occurs when a microbe invades a body and replicates there. Thus, infection needs two things: a body and a microbe. This book explains how certain conditions in the body open the door to infection. Since infection is a normal part of biology, I'll begin my discussion where all discussions in biology begin: the microbe.

Microbes and Microbiology

Infectious organisms are of five types: bacteria, protozoa, fungi, viruses, and parasites (worms, insects, etc.). You will also hear the term *infectious agents* used for these organisms.

Microbiologists study only the microscopic infectious agents, which are organisms that can be seen only by using a microscope.

These microorganisms, microbes for short, are bacteria, protozoa, fungi, and viruses. Parasites, by comparison, are gargantuan and rarely need a microscope to be spotted in water, soil, or food. Parasitologists specialize in these organisms, which will not be covered in-depth here.

Microbes are tiny, but the world of microbiology is huge. Microbes cover every surface on Earth and even live miles underground and in the deepest oceans. The air is full of millions upon millions of microbes.

Because of the diversity of microbes, microbiologists divide their work by specializing in a certain type. For instance, bacteriologists study bacteria, virologists study viruses, mycologists specialize in fungi, and protozoologists focus on protozoa.

Infection Vocabulary

Medical terminology can be confusing and some terms differ only by fine points of definition. Infection is an establishment of a reproducing colony of microbes in a host. A host can be any body, either plant or animal. Some microbes can even be infected by others. *Disease* is a loosely-used word for any condition in which the body changes from its normal condition of health. Although we use this term often, *disease* itself can be difficult to define. Is a cold that lasts three days a disease or is it merely an infection? Not surprisingly, the terms *infection* and *disease* are sometimes used interchangeably.

Pathology focuses on the host; it is the study of how disease changes a body. The term *pathogenesis* focuses on an infecting microbe. It refers to the microbe's activities that create disease in the body.

Toxicity is an illness caused by a toxin, which is a naturally produced poison. Many infectious microbes produce toxins and often the toxin does more damage to the body than the microbe.

Infection and Disease Basics

We know infection is bad, but remember also that infections range from mild to very severe. So there is more to infection than the ability of a few microbes to settle in your body and grow there.

A simple, or localized infection, is the best kind you can get. A few microbes enter the body, multiply for a while, and then the body's defenses spring into action and wipe out these interlopers. At worst, you'll get some redness around the infection and a little tenderness or pain. The body rids itself of infection with a minimal amount of help from you, perhaps a bandage, a drop of antiseptic, and a clean infection site.

Infection turns into infectious disease if either one of two things happens. One is if the infection is left unattended. More dirt might enter the infection site and overwhelm the body's defenses. This increases the chance of the infection spreading deeper into the body. The other likely way to get infectious disease is to be infected by a highly virulent microbe.

Virulence is the ability of a microbe to cause disease. High virulence, such as that of the Ebola virus, means serious disease is likely; low virulence, such as found in cold viruses, means disease might not occur or will be mild if it does occur.

Microbes known to cause disease are always called pathogens and from now on I'll refer to them by that name.

So infection is not the same as disease, and infection does not necessarily turn into a disease every time. A disease is any malfunctioning of a body system, organ, or tissue.

Infection Vocabulary

Tissue is a group of cells of the same type, like skin. An organ is a body part that has a single main function, such as the pancreas. A system is a collection of organs that work together, such as the digestive system.

How many infectious diseases plague humanity? (The plague is one of them! It's caused by the *Yersinia* bacteria carried by rats and spread by fleas.) About 220 pathogens infect humans. To get a handle on infectious disease, it is sometimes easier to think of these diseases in groups rather than by the individual pathogen that causes them. The different infectious disease categories are:

> ➤ Intestinal diseases, including food-borne and waterborne illnesses
> ➤ Tuberculosis (TB)
> ➤ Sexually transmitted diseases (STDs)
> ➤ Non-STD chlamydia diseases

➤ Spirochete bacterial diseases (spirochetes are corkscrew-shaped bacteria)

➤ Rickettsial diseases (rickettsia live inside other cells)

➤ Zoonotic bacterial diseases (diseases that start in animals)

➤ Non-zoonotic bacterial diseases (any disease not listed above)

➤ Viral infections of the central nervous system

➤ Viral infections of skin and mucous membranes

➤ Viral hepatitis (infection of the liver)

➤ Arthropod-borne viral fevers (infections carried by insects)

➤ Human immunodeficiency virus (HIV)

➤ Other viral diseases (any viral disease not listed above)

➤ Mycoses (fungus-caused diseases)

➤ Protozoal diseases

➤ Helminthiases (intestinal worm infections)

➤ Acariasis (mite infestation) and pediculosis (louse infestation)

The last two belong to the realm of parasitologists.

At the Doctor's Office

A person with an infection or disease usually notices certain signs and symptoms of illness. A sign is any objective change in the body, such as a rash, redness, or fever. A symptom is a subjective change, such as loss of appetite, weakness, or dizziness.

When a sick person visits a physician, the doctor examines the patient and usually detects many of the same signs an observant patient might detect. The doctor gathers information on symptoms by asking the patient, "How do you feel?"

The first step toward an accurate diagnosis relies on giving your doctor a complete picture of those subjective feelings of nausea, dizziness, fatigue, chills, etc. Those subjective clues are symptoms of disease.

In general, a sign is something a doctor observes or measures and a symptom is something that a patient perceives.

Infection means good news and bad news. Sooner or later, everyone gets an infection. Because microbes are everywhere, we cannot avoid them. This is the bad news that germophobes fear! But the good news is that only a small percentage of all microbes on Earth are pathogens. Let's meet them.

A Primer on Microbes

Microbes are scary things. We know them as germs. They are invisible on us and on everything we touch, and they have the ability to kill us. No wonder an occasional bestselling book or popular movie uses a germ as the protagonist's diabolical nemesis!

Germ is a nonscientific term for any microbe that causes us trouble by making us sick or spoiling our food. But germs also provide an enormous service: they decompose organic matter. (Organic matter is anything containing the element carbon. For example, protein is organic; granite is inorganic.) Without the microbes in nature, we would be buried in wastes.

In humans, the most common causes of infection are viruses, bacteria, fungi, and yeasts. Protozoa and parasites cause fewer infections in the United States and other developed countries than these four groups. The rarest infectious agent is not even a microbe but a strand of infectious protein called a prion.

Microbe Basics

Bacteria, yeast cells, fungal spores, and most protozoa are invisible to the naked eye. Microbiologists view bacteria (ranging from 0.1 micrometer, or micron (μ) to 10 μ in diameter), yeasts (about 100 μ), spores (50 μ–150 μ), and protozoa (30 μ–300 μ)) under light microscopes. These are the basic microscopes people see in doctors' offices and on TV cop shows. Viruses measure only about 20 to 60 nanometers (nm). Only expensive, complex electron microscopes are capable of making images of viruses.

One μ is a millionth of a meter, or about 0.00004 inch. One nm is a billionth of a meter, or about 0.00000004 inch.

Bacteria

The world of microbes seems to begin with bacteria. Bacteria are single cells that live independently. They were the first organisms on Earth from which everything else evolved. Think about that for a moment. Oak trees, alligators, geraniums, people, and any other living thing you can imagine all started with a bacterial cell about 3.5 billion years ago.

So numerous are bacteria on Earth that they are impossible to count. The human body has so many bacteria on and in it, that if we were to grind ourselves up (apologies for the grisly image) and analyze the DNA, we would appear more bacterial than human!

Considering how many bacteria are all around us, there seems no mystery as to where we get bacterial infections. We get them from everywhere: food, water, moisture droplets in air, dust particles, pets, wild animals, other people. We also pick up a large number of bacteria each time we touch inanimate items such as doorknobs, refrigerator handles, telephones, airplane tray tables—you name it.

Bacteria are prokaryotes, the simplest of all organisms. They're protected in nature by a thick cell wall enforced by a netlike substance called peptidoglycan. The amount of peptidoglycan in the cell wall helps microbiologists divide bacteria into two groups. These groups are based on a staining technique invented in 1884 by the Danish microbiologist Christian Gram. The aptly named Gram stain makes bacteria either gram-negative or gram-positive. These two categories give critical clues to clinical microbiologists in hospitals and help doctors diagnose disease. Stained cells are easier to find in a patient's sample (blood, throat swab, etc.) than unstained microbes. In a microscope, gram-negative cells appear pink and gram-positive cells appear dark blue to purple.

Microbe Basics

Biology contains simple cells, called prokaryotes, and more complex cells, called eukaryotes.

Two types of prokaryotes exist: bacteria and archaea. Archaea look like bacteria in a microscope but differ slightly in composition. Archaea also tend to live in out-of-the-way places like in deep sediments, hot springs, and acid runoff from mines. The best news for us is that archaea cause no known infections.

Protozoa, fungi, yeasts, and algae are eukaryotes. Eukaryotic cells have more complex structures inside them and make up all other living things from honey bees to elephants, mosses to giant redwoods.

Both gram-positive and gram-negative pathogens exist, and neither type is more infectious than the other. The Gram stain offers a clue toward identifying the cause of an infection. For example, gram-positive cocci (round cells) in a throat swab give a strong indication of strep throat, caused by the gram-positive bacterium *Streptococcus*.

I would soon run out of space here if I tried to list all the bacterial infections or diseases known today. The following is a short list of examples:

➤ Acne (*Propionibacterium acnes*)

➤ Strep throat (*Streptococcus*)

➤ Toxic shock syndrome (*Staphylococcus aureus*)

➤ Legionnaires' disease (*Legionella pneumophila*)

➤ Lyme disease (*Borrelia burgdorferi*)

➤ Tuberculosis (*Mycobacterium tuberculosis*)

The most familiar of all bacteria also causes a variety of infections. This pathogen is *Escherichia coli*. (Microbiologists identify a microbe by its genus name followed by its species name and usually abbreviate the genus, thus *E. coli*. If I were a bacterium, I'd be *Maczulak anne* or *M. anne*.) *E. coli* causes gastrointestinal and urinary tract infections. *E. coli* gastroenteritis appears in the news with alarming frequency.

Infections in History

Typhoid Mary was a real person named Mary Mallon who cooked for well-to-do New York City families between 1896 and 1906. During this time, typhoid fever was a constant threat in the densely-populated tenements of large cities. Many cases were linked to drinking water contaminated with the fecal bacterium *Salmonella typhi*. Although Mary Mallon did not cause the typhoid scare of the 1900s, she played a prominent role in its history.

Astute New York public health officials noticed that at least twenty-eight typhoid cases occurred in households where Mallon worked. Although they arrested Mallon and she promised never to work again as a cook, upon her release from isolation on an island in New York's East River, she changed her name and again took to the stove, this time at a hospital. New cases of typhoid soon appeared, yet Mary escaped the law for another five years. Authorities tracked down Mary and again deported her to an isolated cell, where she remained for twenty-three years until her death in 1938.

Dubbed Typhoid Mary by journalists, Mallon was bitter at her treatment and never accepted that she had caused any illnesses because she claimed, correctly, she had never been sick. Stool samples in fact proved that Mary was an asymptomatic carrier of *S. typhi*. Ten outbreaks of typhoid fever, more than fifty individual cases, and at least three deaths were attributed to her. Many more may have occurred that officials could never trace back to Mary but were probably caused by her.

As part of the Typhoid Mary experience, doctors learned more about asymptomatic carriers and the manner in which food-borne illness spreads.

Many factors combine to cause food-borne infections, but, as in the case of *E. coli* gastroenteritis, the main culprit is poor hygiene. Put bluntly, a food preparer unwittingly contaminates food with feces. Since domesticated and wild animals also shed *E. coli* in their feces, any meat or crop contaminated with manure or dirty water has the potential to cause food-borne infection. It doesn't take much: a chunk of dried feces half the size of the tip of your pinkie finger carries billions of *E. coli* cells plus other pathogens.

Protozoa

Protozoa are several times larger than bacteria. Unlike bacteria, many protozoa have fragile outer walls that make them vulnerable in the environment. This partially explains why protozoa stay in watery locales, such as freshwater ponds, marine waters, and the digestive tract.

The most famous of protozoa may be the amoeba, a cell of ever-changing shape that creeps through its environment like an otherworldly creature. The *Entamoeba histolytica* amoeba should indeed be feared because it's the cause of the nasty amoebic dysentery.

You may not be as familiar with the most common protozoal infections, but if you spend lots of time camping in the backcountry or traveling to the tropics, you should know these:

➤ Giardiasis (*Giardia lamblia*)

➤ Cryptosporidiosis (*Cryptosporidium*)

➤ Malaria (*Plasmodium*)

➤ Leishmaniasis (*Leishmania*)

➤ Toxoplasmosis (*Toxoplasma gondii*)

➤ Chagas' disease (*Trypanosoma cruzi*)

➤ African sleeping sickness or trypanosomiasis (*Trypanosoma brucei*)

➤ Trichomoniasis (*Trichomonas vaginalis*), an STD

Fungi

Fungi are common in nature, especially in soil, and include yeasts and molds. Yeast is a fungus that lives as a single cell. Mold is a fungus that produces fuzzy or filamentous growth on foods, leather, and clothing. Most everyone is familiar with mold. Just toss a slice of bread onto the kitchen counter and go away for summer vacation. When you return, you can begin a new career in mycology!

Some fungi assemble into multicellular organisms that grow so large they can be seen without a microscope. Bread mold, the mildew in bathrooms, and mushrooms offer examples of organisms that hardly can be called microscopic. Mildew is similar to mold. *Mildew* is a general term for any mold growing in a thin, fuzzy, or matted sheet over an object's surface. Leather, clothes, handbags, books, and plastics often have mildew if left undisturbed for long periods. Mildew does not usually infect humans.

As I mentioned, a single fungus can grow to massive dimensions by adding material to stringy filaments (hyphae) until it makes a tangle or fuzz called a mycelium. The largest known organism on Earth is an underground fungus in eastern Oregon's Blue Mountains. This mushroom called *Armillaria ostoyae* covers 2,384 acres, equivalent to 1,665 football fields. *A. ostoyae*'s hyphae infect conifer roots and kill many of the trees in its path.

Fungal infection occurs on a much smaller scale in humans, of course, but the human pathogens work in much the same way as *A. ostoyae*, by secreting enzymes that digest tissue.

Examples of fungal infections or diseases are:

➤ Tinea pedis (athlete's foot; *Trichophyton*)

➤ Tinea cruris (jock itch; *Trichophyton*)

➤ Pneumocystis pneumonia (*Pneumocystis jiroveci*)

➤ Histoplasmosis (*Histoplasma capsulatum*)

Airborne fungi also cause allergies and the ailment known as sick building syndrome. The main fungi involved in these illnesses are: *Aspergillus*, *Cladosporium*, *Mucor*, *Penicillium*, and *Stachybotrys*.

The most common yeast infection is candidiasis caused by *Candida albicans*. This species infects the mucous membranes of the genitourinary tract and the mouth, where the infection is called thrush. Other yeast infections are:

➤ Cryptococcosis (*Cryptococcus neoformans* and *C. gattii*)

➤ Folliculitis (*Malassezia furfur*)

➤ Dandruff (*M. furfur*)

Algae

Most people have an idea of what algae are, but they may not be able to pinpoint the specifics of algae or name even one member of this huge group of organisms. Hint: kelp forests in the ocean and green growth in a spa are both algae. Yes, it's a very diverse group of organisms.

Algae usually live in water and lack leaves, stems, and roots. Most important, algae perform photosynthesis, which makes these organisms vital to life on Earth. Only photosynthetic organisms (green plants, algae, and bacteria called cyanobacteria) convert the sun's energy into chemical energy that fuels every other living thing.

The main health threat from algae comes from the toxins several species excrete. Algal toxins are called neurotoxins because they affect the nervous system; they will be discussed in Chapter 5.

Viruses

Viral infections have always been part of human history. Viruses infect animal cells, plant cells, and bacteria, and they are usually very specific to the type of cell they infect. In other words, a virus that attacks trees would not be expected to infect humans. But biology is full of exceptions. The most notable example of a virus that attacks more than one species is influenza, nicknamed the flu. The flu virus infects chickens, ducks, and other birds, as well as swine, before jumping to humans.

Viruses employ a stealthy scheme of infiltrating a host cell, and then commandeering the cell's replication to make more viruses. When you catch a cold, cells lining your nasal passages build an assembly plant for producing thousands of new cold viruses. This assembly plant snaps into action after no more than thirty minutes after the first cold virus comes in contact with the mucous membranes inside the nose. Little wonder that computer experts coined the term *virus* to mean an electronic bug that enters the host (your computer) and uses the host's own systems for making and spreading more viruses.

To make our battles against viruses all the more complicated, virus infections can be acute, latent, or persistent. Acute infections develop quickly and lead to a relatively short period of disease, such as a cold or the flu. Latent infections hide in the body for long periods—years to decades—without causing disease symptoms. The herpes virus, human immunodeficiency virus (HIV, the cause of acquired immunodeficiency syndrome, or AIDS), and chickenpox (varicella-zoster viruses) cause latent infections.

Viruses produce more diseases than any other type of pathogen.

The following are examples of viral infections in humans:

➤ Common cold (rhinovirus)

➤ Influenza or flu (influenza virus)

➤ Chickenpox (varicella-zoster virus)

➤ Measles (rubella virus)

➤ Hepatitis (hepatitis A, B, C, D, or E virus)

➤ Viral gastroenteritis, or stomach flu (rotavirus and norovirus)

➤ Herpes (herpes simplex virus)

➤ Sudden acute respiratory syndrome, or SARS (coronavirus)

➤ Rabies (rabies virus)

Infections and Disease

Infectious diseases can be communicable and contagious. A communicable disease is one in which a pathogen has been transmitted from one host to another, such as from one person to another person, from one animal to a person, or from a person to an animal.

Some communicable diseases are also contagious diseases, meaning they move from host to host by direct or close contact. Thus, sexually transmitted diseases and influenza are contagious; food-borne illnesses are not contagious.

Frank Pathogens versus Opportunistic Pathogens

Germophobes beware. Though the microbial world contains relatively few pathogens, many of the harmless microbes also turn into pathogens if the right opportunity presents itself.

Microbiologists divide pathogens into the proven disease causers and the microbes that need a little nudge. A frank pathogen is a microbe that has been proven to cause disease following infection. For example, tuberculosis is caused by a frank pathogen. An opportunistic pathogen, by contrast, will not normally cause infection unless conditions in the host change to favor an infection.

Normal Flora and Opportunists

The normal flora of your body includes up to four hundred different species living on the skin, in the respiratory tract, and in the digestive tract. Most are bacteria, but we also harbor smaller numbers of fungi (on skin) and protozoa (in the intestines). Many species are found on everyone but, like a fingerprint, we also host a unique mixture of species.

Most of the time normal flora stays where it's supposed to stay. *Staphylococcus aureus* (sometimes called *Staph aureus*) normally resides in the nasal passages, where it causes no harm. But if a person gets a cut or wound, the *Staph aureus* might find its way into that wound and start an infection. When this happens, *Staph aureus* has gone from being a member of the normal flora to being an opportunistic pathogen.

Staph aureus may be the champion of opportunistic pathogens because it possesses a quality called invasiveness. An invasive pathogen can spread from an infection site to other tissues. This is why a *Staph aureus* infection that starts on the skin can lead to pneumonia (lungs), mastitis (breast tissue), endocarditis (heart), osteomyelitis (bone), sepsis (blood), or gastroenteritis. *Staph aureus* is truly an all-purpose pathogen.

Not all opportunistic pathogens come from your normal flora. Many opportunists are fungi, bacteria, and protozoa that come from your surroundings.

At the Doctor's Office

Nosocomial infections arise from pathogens that are more prevalent in hospitals than they are in nonmedical places. In addition to hospitals, nosocomial infections originate in outpatient clinics, doctors' and dentists' offices, dialysis clinics, and long-term care facilities. The Centers for Disease Control and Prevention (CDC) now refers to these as healthcare-associated infections (HAI) because of the various medical facilities where the pathogens exist.

About a decade ago, more than 10 percent of all hospital patients acquired an HAI. Today, special efforts by the medical community have helped reduce HAIs significantly. Still, in a confined environment where people are weakened by disease and other infections, and where antibiotic use has created resistant strains, hospitals are prime places for picking up dangerous germs.

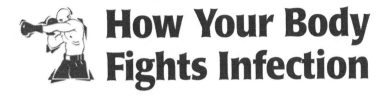

CHAPTER 2

How Your Body Fights Infection

In This Chapter

➤ The main components of the body's defense system

➤ The body's immovable defenses against infection

➤ Immunity, the body's responsive defense against infection

➤ The basics of innate defense

➤ How the body's immune system is organized

➤ Comparing nonspecific and specific immune components

➤ Features of a host that contribute to infection

In this chapter you will see the ways the body defends itself against infection. These defenses are critical for survival and yet they happen without your knowledge. A person would not live to old age without the basic static defenses as well as defenses that can change and respond to different types of germs. To put their importance in perspective, humanity would not have made it this far without its defenses against germs having evolved right along with us.

The body's germ defense has two characteristics to assure the best possible fortress against invasion. Biologists call these characteristics redundancy and duality.

Redundancy means that more than one process is available to do the same job. If one type of defense fails, a second should be up to the task and kill the pathogen. For example, if the skin is injured and can't stop germs, specialized cells in the bloodstream rush into action to kill invading microbes.

Duality means that the body's immunity is built on two separate but complementary systems that work in different ways toward the same goal: stopping infection. Like redundancy, duality ensures that if a pathogen bypasses one defense, a second type of defense might work better to stop it.

Best of all, your defenses work behind the scenes, fighting off pathogens several times a day without your knowledge. All that you have to do to help them is to have a healthy diet, get plenty of rest, and reduce stress.

The Body's Defenses Against Infection

The body's defenses consist of organs, tissues, and a dizzying variety of cell types. These components can be hard to keep straight. And why should you if the system works without your active participation, like heartbeats or digestion do? In this chapter, I'll highlight the main components of infection defense. By understanding the body's defenses, you learn the basics of fighting infection. All barriers to infection are collectively referred to as host resistance.

Host resistance has two components: innate defenses and the immune system, or immunity. The innate component consists of all-purpose barriers to invasion such as skin. By contrast, the immune system is much more specific. Immunity begins developing in early childhood. Its purpose is to respond to specific infectious agents with equally specific reactions. Furthermore, the immune system provides both short-term protection against infection and long-term protection. After infection by certain pathogens, the body's immune system can protect you against that same pathogen for the rest of your life.

Your Body, a Host for Infectious Agents

The object of the game in fighting infection is to resist any microbe that has the potential to cause harm to bodily tissues. As you've seen, a pathogen is a microbe that causes disease. By definition, this also means that pathogens harm the body for their own benefit. Another name for pathogen is parasite.

Host resistance tries to fight off infection from the first contact of a pathogen with the body to the deepest infiltrations of parasites inside tissues and organs.

Innate Defenses

Innate defense, or innate resistance, is your body on autopilot for fighting infection. These defenses are the physical, chemical, or biological factors that you are born with or develop early in life.

The physical barriers against infection, such as skin, represent a first line of defense. This defensive line is the first thing a pathogen encounters when it finds you and sizes you up as a potential host. After the first line of defense, biological and chemical factors give the host a second line of defense.

Physical Barriers in Innate Defense

The body puts up three physical barriers to infection: the skin, mucous membranes, and the tiny cilia (hairlike projections) lining parts of the respiratory tract.

Infection Vocabulary

Epithelium consists of a layer of cells that form the outer layer of skin and the surface layer of mucous membranes. Sometimes the epithelium contains a single layer of cells and in other instances it consists of several layers. Specialized epithelial cells also exist so that the body has some that hold tiny hairs called cilia or possess activity like glands do.

Connective tissue is one of the body's four basic cell types. (The others are epithelium, nerve, and muscle.) Connective tissue gives the body an underlying structure upon which epithelium lies. It also serves to hold together muscle tissue and nervous tissue. Unlike epithelium, connective tissue cells do not have to be directly connected to each other.

Healthy, intact skin forms the strongest defense against invasion. The skin, or epidermis, is a large organ. The human body is covered by about 6.5 square feet of skin, which also carries several of the biological and chemical components of the second defensive line, the immune system.

The skin itself has two main layers and is more complex than it looks at first glance. Each layer acts differently as a barrier against infection:

➤ Epidermis: Thin outermost layer of skin that contains mainly dead skin cells and the tough, protective protein keratin.

➤ Dermis: Thicker inner layer of reproducing skin cells, connective tissue, and a blood supply that delivers specialized substances from the immune system.

Like skin, mucous membranes contain epithelial cells and an underlying layer of connective tissue. These membranes cover the entire inner lining of the digestive tract (mouth to anus), respiratory tract, and genitourinary tracts.

Mucous membranes secrete a thick, fluid called mucus. (*Mucous* is an adjective and *mucus* is a noun.) Mucus prevents the tracts from drying out, which is important because pathogens cross dry membranes easier than they cross moist, intact membranes. Mucous membranes do not protect the body as well as skin does. These membranes are in fact favorite sites upon which pathogens attach to the body and gain entry.

Another physical pathogen-repelling mechanism works in the respiratory tract. Hairs inside the nose trap many particles and filter inhaled air. In addition, cells lining the lower respiratory tract have tiny cilia (very fine hairlike projections) that beat in coordinated waves. These waves push particles toward the throat and away from the lungs. The waves comprise the ciliary escalator, capable of propelling particles out of the body at a rate of about an inch an hour.

Infection Vocabulary

A substance's pH tells you about its level of acidity. Specifically, pH refers to the concentration of hydrogen molecules (H^+), and acids have a very high concentration of H^+.

Every liquid in the environment has a pH. The pH scale extends from 0, the most acidic, to 14, the most basic, or alkaline. A pH of 7.0 means a material is neutral; it is neither acidic nor basic. As a reference, lemon juice is pH 2, milk is pH 6.8, and soap is pH 10. Human skin is slightly acidic, about pH 5.

Chemical Factors in Innate Defense

The body has a variety of chemicals that inhibit foreign microbes. Chemicals on the skin include sebum, acidic fats, sweat, and digestive enzymes. Sweat helps flush away some infectious agents and also contains the enzyme lysozyme, which degrades the outer cell wall of bacteria. Tears, saliva, nasal secretions, and some tissue secretions also contain lysozyme.

In the stomach, gastric juice produces extremely acidic

conditions, with almost the same acidity as battery acid! A microbe that enters the stomach is likely to be killed on contact.

If an infectious agent manages to make it all the way to the intestines, it confronts more chemical warfare produced by the body. Digestive enzymes secreted by the intestines can digest microbial cells. At the same time, bile stored in the gallbladder also inhibits microbial growth. Finally, the intestines eject infectious agents via peristalsis. Peristalsis consists of pulse-like waves of the intestinal wall that move solid matter toward the exit, the anus.

Biological Factors in Innate Defense

One type of biological defense called bacteriocins comes from your body's normal flora. The other type is a white blood cell that comes from your immune system.

Bacteriocins are like antibiotics. Your normal flora produces bacteriocins to repel other microbes that shouldn't be on your skin or in your digestive tract.

Microbe Basics

Bacteriocins are like antibiotics; they are substances produced by one microbe to kill another microbe. Microbiologists make a slight distinction between bacteriocins and antibiotics. Microbes make antibiotics to kill unrelated microbes; bacteriocins kill closely related microbes. For example, the antibiotic penicillin made by the fungus *Penicillium* kills bacteria. The bacteriocin called staphylococcin made by *Staphylococcus* kills other strains of *Staphylococcus*. Bacteriocins help the normal flora defend its home, the host's body, against foreign invaders, even when the foreigners are cousins!

The second biological factor is a white blood cell called phagocyte. First, let's take a look at blood. Like wine, blood can be divided into two basic types: red and white. Red blood cells carry oxygen and make clots. Blood clots play an important part in infection control by sealing off infection sites and protecting the rest of the body from invasion by pathogens. White blood cells include many different types that have diverse roles in fighting infection.

Phagocytes are very flexible; they move through the circulatory system and tissues as if they were amoebae. When a phagocyte comes upon a particle that doesn't belong in the body, it engulfs it and then digests it. This process is called phagocytosis.

Phagocytosis is an example of redundancy because more than one type of phagocyte can do it. The body's main phagocytes are:

> ➤ Neutrophils: Destroy pathogens in the early stages of infection

> ➤ Eosinophils: Destroy protozoa in the early stages of infection

> ➤ Macrophages: White blood cells that wander freely in blood and tissue, destroying any foreign particles.

At the Doctor's Office

Doctors gather a lot of clues about your health by examining the relative numbers of red and white blood cells after you give a blood sample. Abnormalities in the white blood cell (WBC) count indicate the presence of an infection.

Normal ranges for the WBC test are:

> ➤ Total WBC count: 4,500–10,000 per microliter (μL)

> ➤ Eosinophils: Less than 350/ μL or 1–4 percent in the blood

> ➤ Basophils: 0.0–2.0 percent

> ➤ Neutrophils: 40–60 percent

> ➤ Monocytes: 2–8 percent

> ➤ Lymphocytes: 20–40 percent

The percent values of all five types of WBC are called the blood differential.

When all of these cells, except basophils, increase above normal, you probably have an infection.

How the Immune System is Organized

The immune system has organs, tissues, and individual cells that give you a third line of defense against infection. All together they provide you with immunity, which is your overall ability to detect a foreign substance and eliminate it. (Immunology is the study of all aspects of the immune system.)

Biologists divide the immune response into two types. One is a nonspecific type. This nonspecific immunity defends against infections regardless of the particular infectious agent. The other type is specific, or adaptive, immunity. This type consists of components that produce specific responses to particular infectious agents. Both nonspecific and specific are equally crucial to you in fighting infection.

Infection Vocabulary

The lymphatic system consists of all the vessels that carry a fluid called lymph throughout the body. Lymph is a colorless liquid containing immune system proteins, salts, urea, fats and sugar, and cells called lymphocytes and monocytes.

Lymphocytes play multiple necessary roles in the immune system's infection fighting. Particularly, lymphocytes detect the presence of foreign particles in the blood or in body tissue and work in concert with other immune system cells to destroy them.

Monocytes are white blood cells that circulate in the body in search of invaders. They are one of the main cells that do phagocytosis.

Nonspecific Immunity

Nonspecific immunity comes from three types of white blood cells (also called leukocytes): neutrophils, eosinophils, and basophils. You have already seen that the first two perform phagocytosis. Basophils do not carry out phagocytosis but instead release the following battery of chemicals that play a part in inflammation:

➤ Histamine: Dilates blood vessels and increases vessel permeability so immunity substances can reach the infection site

➤ Leukotriene: Constricts vessels, increases permeability, and attracts macrophages to the infection site

➤ Serotonin: Affects vessel dilation and permeability

➤ Prostaglandin: Dilates and constricts vessels and induces pain. (Pain warns the host of infection or other injury.)

Infections and Disease

Inflammation is never fun. With it comes redness, pain, heat, and swelling. Despite your discomfort with these events, inflammation serves an important role in fighting infection. Sometimes an inflammation kills pathogens. In other instances, inflammation can't by itself destroy the infectious agents, but it helps confine them to the infection site so other immune responses can finish the job.

The immune system also uses a mixture of some thirty proteins comprising the complement system. Complement proteins are normally dormant in the blood. The presence of an infectious agent activates one complement, which then starts a cascade of activations of the other complement proteins. The activation may result from substances on the surface of a pathogen, protein called lectin in the bloodstream that binds to pathogen cells, or the binding of antibodies to any foreign substance. An antibody is a specialized protein made by the immune system to destroy specific foreign matter. A fully activated complement system helps in immunity by all of the following activities:

➤ Recruits additional phagocytes

➤ Enhances phagocytosis of bacteria by coating the bacterial cells

➤ Directs attack on pathogens

➤ Mediates inflammation

Infections and Disease

A fever is a body temperature raised above the normal. Fever occurs during some infections when the infectious agent causes a large amount of cytokines to be released by immune system cells and damaged tissue. The cytokines induce the brain to reset the body's thermostat, and they turn on heat-producing mechanisms.

Fever intensifies many of the reactions of the immune system when fighting infection. It may also inhibit the growth of some pathogens and speed up tissue repair. After the infection has been eliminated, the brain returns the thermostat to normal and initiates cooling mechanisms.

During a fever, the body feels hot to the touch, but the sick person may feel chills. In the cooldown period after a fever, the person sweats and is flushed due to dilation of blood vessels, which also helps with cooling.

Temperatures from just over 94° Fahrenheit to 98.6° Fahrenheit are considered normal for people. Hard exercise or infection raises body temperature to a range of 99°F to 104°F. Brain damage or heatstroke can occur at temperatures above 104°F.

Specific Immunity

Remember the duality of the immune system? While nonspecific parts of your immune system are on constant duty, like a sentry at the gate to an army base, trained assault teams are waiting for a chance to spring into action. These assault teams are analogous to your specific immunity.

Specific immunity (also called acquired immunity) is either natural or artificial. Each of these two types can be further divided into two different forms: active and passive.

Natural specific immunity means antibodies. Antibodies are proteins that circulate in the blood and attach to invading substances. Antibodies either destroy the invader or hang onto it until immune system reinforcements arrive to destroy it. Antibodies' claim to fame comes from their very specific connection to an invader, called an antigen. The body assembles antibodies so that they fit perfectly with a given antigen, like a lock and key.

Biologists differentiate between the active and passive forms of natural immunity this way:

➤ Active: An antigen enters the body and the body responds by producing antibodies to bind with that very antigen

➤ Passive: Antibodies for specific antigens pass from a mother to a fetus during gestation or to a nursing infant in mother's milk.

Artificial specific immunity comes in the form of a vaccine. Vaccines contain either antibodies or antigens, and these two choices also determine whether the artificial immunity will be active or passive:

➤ Active: A vaccine contains antigens, which forces the body to produce antibodies against them.

➤ Passive: A vaccine contains pre-formed antibodies.

The Duality of the Immune System

As more and more components of the immune system were discovered throughout the twentieth century and to the present, biologists began to realize that the immune system uses a two-pronged attack against most infections. One prong comes from the action of antibodies. This makes up humoral immunity, or antibody-mediated immunity. The second prong results from the activity of lymphocytes and is thus called cell-mediated immunity. These complementary parts of the immune system are described as follows:

➤ Humoral immunity: Lymphocytes called B cells produce antibodies that circulate and work in blood, lymph fluid, and mucus.

➤ Cell-mediated immunity: Lymphocytes called T cells act alone or regulate the activity of other cells such as macrophages.

Infections and Disease

Why do infectious diseases present a greater hazard to health in poor parts of the world than in affluent societies? Many factors influence the incidence of infection and a community's ability to control an infection's spread.

Poor regions often lack a strong medical infrastructure, which helps doctors and their patients fight infection. In truth, some communities don't have a doctor less than a day's travel away. Impoverished areas also have many, if not all, of the following characteristics:

➤ Malnutrition

➤ Preexisting or chronic disease

➤ Densely-populated communities

➤ Sporadic or improperly tested drug supply

➤ Expired antibiotics

➤ Limited availability of medical attention

Certain impoverished communities in the tropics have high exposure to insects and animals that carry infectious agents, further increasing the chances of being infected.

A Weakened Host Equals Increased Risk of Infection

Pathogens have been around since the earliest recorded history, so we know they have tricks up their proverbial sleeves to outsmart the immune system. Infectious agents are also helped immensely when a host's defenses have been weakened. Like people, pathogens follow a path of least resistance to their goal. A weak immune system signals to a pathogen, "This way!"

Innate defenses against infection are inherited from our parents. Every healthy person has the same basic innate defenses, some a little stronger than the norm and others a little weaker. There is nothing you can do about your genetics.

Specific immunity, by contrast, has been called adaptive immunity because it develops based on a person's experiences. A person living in an apartment in New York City faces a different array of microbes than does a farmer in Iowa. Their immune systems therefore also adapt to the infectious agents of the Big Apple and the Hawkeye State, respectively.

A predisposing factor is any feature of a person that makes him or her more susceptible to infection than other people. Though many of these factors remain unknown, epidemiologists have gathered a lot of information on who is more likely to get an infection compared with the general population. Their research has led to focus mainly on gender, age, climate and weather, personal habits, lifestyle, and occupation.

Almost all people have certain high-risk factors that are part of their life and/or work. These high-risk factors are known to increase the chance of infection:

- ➤ Poor nutrition
- ➤ Fatigue
- ➤ Emotional stress
- ➤ Preexisting illness
- ➤ Chronic disease
- ➤ Old age
- ➤ Very young age
- ➤ Pregnancy
- ➤ Chemotherapy
- ➤ Organ transplantation

A person who has had his or her immune system suppressed by cancer chemotherapy or antirejection drugs used with organ transplantation is called immunocompromised.

Infections and Disease

Dental caries (tooth decay) is a type of infection caused by the formation of a film called plaque over the tooth enamel. Bacteria in plaque digest sugars in food and excrete lactic acid as an end product. The acid in turn begins to degrade the enamel, forming pits, or caries.

Plaque formation follows several steps. Within minutes of brushing teeth, various bacteria begin forming a thin film called pellicle on a clean tooth. Within a couple of hours, different species attach to the pellicle and excrete a gummy polysaccharide called dextran. Other bacteria and food particles soon get trapped in the dextran. Before long, a mixture of polysaccharide, food, saliva, and bacteria covers the tooth, and this mixture is plaque. Of the more than four hundred species of bacteria that make up plaque, the main instigator of caries is lactic acid–producing *Streptococcus mutans*.

Dental caries were uncommon in Western society until about the seventeenth century. The increased popularity of table sugar coincided with a rise in dental caries, and they are now one of our most common infections.

Susceptibility

The word *susceptibility* is the best way to summarize your risk of infection. *Susceptibility* means weak resistance to infection or disease. High susceptibility translates to a high risk for infection; low susceptibility means a person is relatively safe from infection.

Susceptibility to a particular pathogen, such as the flu virus, varies from species to species. For example, both pigs and humans may be susceptible to the same influenza germ, but their susceptibility to a specific flu strain may differ. You probably already know that susceptibility also varies within a species. That is, susceptibility to a given infectious agent varies from person to person.

Gender determines susceptibility to certain germs but not others. For instance, women are more likely than men to contract a urinary tract infection (UTI).

After gender, age is an important indicator of whether a person is at high risk or normal risk of susceptibility. Children under age six and the elderly (sixty-five years or older) have a higher risk of infection because of a weakened immune system. In children, the immune system may not yet be fully formed to fight off certain invaders. In the elderly, immunity is often weakened by a consortium of factors. Often a factor in elder infection is the presence of other underlying chronic diseases.

At the Doctor's Office

Certain types of cancer increase a person's chance of infection. The chemotherapy or radiation therapy used to treat cancer also suppresses the body's immune system. These conditions lower the total number of a person's white blood cells as well as other immune system cells that fight infections.

Doctors monitor a cancer patient's WBC, especially neutrophils. A low number of neutrophils, a condition called neutropenia, indicates that the patient has an increased risk of infection. Doctors base their conclusion on a value called the absolute neutrophil count (ANC), which should be 50–70 percent of total white blood cells. An ANC of less than 1,000 means neutrophils are low and the immune system is weak. ANCs of 500 or lower put a person at very high risk of serious infection.

Genetics also plays a role in susceptibility. For example, Native Americans and Asians are more susceptible to the tuberculosis pathogen (*Mycobacterium tuberculosis*) than are

Caucasians. Similarly, the inherited trait that produces sickle-cell anemia is higher in people whose ancestors come from sub-Saharan Africa, Saudi Arabia, India, and parts of the Mediterranean and Spanish-speaking regions, than it is in the rest of the population. The sickle-cell trait is carried by one in twelve African Americans. Sometimes the same genetics that play a role in susceptibility have a beneficial effect. The sickle-cell trait makes individuals resistant to the protozoan that causes malaria (various species of *Plasmodium*).

Susceptibility alone does not doom a person to infection and disease. For any infection to happen, a potential host must be exposed to an infectious agent. Remember too that infectious agents cover a huge range in their ability to infect and cause disease.

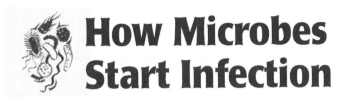

CHAPTER 3

How Microbes Start Infection

In This Chapter

➤ The meaning of virulence and the main virulence factors

➤ The features that change a harmless microbe into a pathogen

➤ How pathogens evade a body's defenses

➤ The main target tissues of common pathogens

➤ Introduction to the major infectious diseases and their causes

In this chapter you will learn the clever ways used by microbes to get around the body's three lines of defense against infection. So diabolical are pathogens, many have devised tactics that use the body itself to help spread infection. The most insidious invaders, such as the AIDS virus, invade the body's immune system, the very system intended to fight infection.

Infection can occur only if three things are present: a pathogen, a host, and a way to transmit the pathogen to the host. The previous chapter described the main parts of a host's defense against infection. This chapter focuses on the pathogen. It begins with pathogenicity, the ability of a microbe to cause disease by overcoming a host's defenses.

Pathogenicity

Microbes possess certain features on their cells that determine whether they will be pathogenic or nonpathogenic. Among the pathogenic microbes, certain features determine the intensity of the disease they cause. These features are called virulence factors. A pathogen with high virulence causes serious disease; a pathogen with low virulence causes less serious disease.

The most-studied virulence factors are:

> ➤ Infectivity: Ability of a microbe to establish an initial infection

> ➤ Invasiveness: Ability of the microbe to spread to other tissues

> ➤ Pathogenic potential: Degree to which the pathogen causes damage to the host

> ➤ Toxigenicity: Ability of the pathogen to produce toxins, which are chemicals that damage the body's tissues

> ➤ Infectious dose: Dose or number of pathogens needed to start an infection

> ➤ Lethal dose: Dose or number of pathogens needed to kill a host

At the Doctor's Office

The CDC is this country's national resource for health issues. Your doctor keeps track of the latest news on infectious agents and disease outbreaks by reading current medical literature and by checking the CDC's news and resources.

The CDC consists of several centers that focus on particular areas of personal or public health. The CDC's Office of Infectious Diseases provides resources on all the subjects in this book.

Different microbes can differ markedly in these six virulence factors. The right combination makes each known pathogen on Earth more or less able to cause infection and disease. For example, let's compare the infectious dose of two food-borne pathogens, *Salmonella* and *Shigella*. *Salmonella* needs a fairly high infectious dose of from about 100 to 1,000 cells to cause infection. *Shigella* can infect with only 10 or so cells present in a food. In addition, *Shigella*'s toxigenicity is very high; *Salmonella*'s is lower. As a result, *Shigella*'s virulence is higher than *Salmonella*'s virulence, yet both are pathogens and both can kill a host with a weak immune system.

What makes a microbe a pathogen? And what turns a run-of-the-mill pathogen into a dangerous, life-threatening pathogen? The answers lie in how well a microbe has adapted to the host's defenses. The most virulent pathogens possess mechanisms that trick, perplex, and evade the host's immune system, as well as cause serious damage to tissues. Often bacteria, fungi, protozoa, and viruses have developed their own set of tactics for evading host defenses and damaging host tissue.

The objectives of any pathogen are to enter the host, move around in the host to find a favorite type of tissue (the target tissue or organ), replicate, and exit the host so the pathogen can find new hosts to infect.

Infections in History

Koch's postulates consists of principles by which a given pathogen could be connected to a specific disease in humans. Developed by German physician and microbiologist Robert Koch (pronounced like coke) in the mid-1880s, these principles built the framework for today's diagnosis of infectious disease.

The postulates are:

➤ A microbe must be present in every case of a disease but absent from a healthy individual.

➤ The microbe must be isolated from a sick person and grown in a laboratory.

➤ The same disease should result if the microbe were to be put into a healthy individual.

➤ The same microbe must be re-isolated from the diseased individual.

These postulates were tested on laboratory animals rather than humans.

How Pathogens Enter a Host

The first step in infection involves the attachment of a microbe to the host. The attachment occurs either on the skin or on a mucous membrane. This step is called contact.

The point of entry into the host is called a portal of entry. Pathogens often cannot penetrate healthy, intact skin, but they can penetrate skin that has been injured by a cut, scratch, puncture, burn, rash, or any other circumstance that disrupts the normal skin layers.

Mucous membranes present a more inviting portal of entry to many pathogens. The cells of mucous membranes are not as tightly packed as skin cells and the moisture inherent in mucous membranes also helps the pathogen. Even intact healthy mucous membranes fail to defend against certain viruses, food-borne bacteria, airborne pathogens, and sexually transmitted diseases. The mucous membranes most vulnerable to infection occur in the gastrointestinal, respiratory, urinary, and genital tracts, and the conjunctiva of the eye.

Once pathogens establish a small beachhead at the infection site, they have two options: build a colony there or spread to another part of the body. The cold virus (rhinovirus) stays at its initial entry site in the upper respiratory tract and causes all its damage right there. By contrast, the sexually transmitted AIDS virus (HIV) spreads from its initial entry site at the mucous membranes of the vagina or the rectum to the bloodstream. The bloodstream then carries HIV to nervous tissue and cells of the immune system.

How Bacterial Pathogens Evade Host Defenses

Bacteria have various strategies for fighting off the host's defenses during the first critical stages of establishing an infection. Most people (who are neither microbiologists nor germophobes) fight off several potential infections every week. We ingest pathogens with meals, get dirt in a skin wound, and rub grime into our eyes. Adults in fact touch the mucous membranes of the face (eyes, mouth, and nose) with their hands dozens of times a day. Children do it hundreds of times a day. With each touch comes a likely dose of microbes with perhaps a small percentage of frank pathogens. In healthy people with a strong immune system, the body annihilates the infectious microbes swiftly and efficiently.

Microbe Basics

Enzymes are the substances secreted by microbes to do microbial jobs. In infection, pathogens release enzymes to break down connective tissue to expand the infection site, to clot the blood surrounding an infection site, to destroy substances meant to kill them (such as antibiotics), and to get nutrients from the host's body.

In some cases, the balance tips in favor of the pathogen. Maybe the host's defenses have been already weakened by a cold or a person ingests a very high dose of pathogen cells. Perhaps you are unlucky enough to come in contact with a very virulent pathogen. Once inside the body, the most devious of virulent pathogens pull from their bag of tricks some of the following ways to evade the body's immune response:

➤ Capsules: Outer coating made of polysaccharide prevents destruction by the body's phagocytosis system (Example: *Streptococcus pneumoniae*, the cause of pneumonia.)

➤ M Proteins: Protein on the bacterial cell's surface helps it bind tightly to the host epithelial cells and avoid phagocytosis. (Example: *Streptococcus pyogenes*, the cause of toxic shock syndrome and necrotizing fasciitis.)

➤ Enzymes: Proteins secreted by bacteria that neutralize the blood's immune factors. (Example: *Staphylococcus aureus* makes the enzyme coagulase, which clots the blood around an infection site, protecting the pathogen from other host factors in the bloodstream.)

➤ Serum resistance factors: Production of specialized polysaccharides on the bacterial cell surface that interferes with the host's normal complement system in fighting infection. (Example: *Neisseria gonorrhoeae*, the cause of gonorrhea, activates its resistance factors to allow it to spread unhindered through the bloodstream.)

Avoiding Phagocytosis

The objective of most pathogens in the early stage of infection is to avoid being eaten by a phagocyte. Bacteria have evolved various ways of circumventing phagocytosis aside from the formation of a capsule. The tuberculosis pathogen *Mycobacterium* builds a waxy outer coat that resists phagocytosis. If a persistent phagocyte manages to engulf the *Mycobacterium* cell, the waxy layer prevents digestion by the phagocyte's enzymes.

Other bacteria, such as *Shigella*, *Rickettsia*, and *Listeria*, play hide-and-seek inside the phagocyte. These bacteria take special care to avoid the lysosome. A lysosome is a sac inside each phagocyte that contains all the enzymes the phagocyte needs for digesting bacteria. The pathogens that hide inside host cells quickly swim to the phagocyte's outer surface. From there, they escape before the phagocyte can release the deadly enzymes, often jumping to other phagocytes!

Bacteria, like viruses and some protozoa, also have a feature called antigenic variation. Antigenic variation allows a pathogen to alter the substances on the outside of its cell. This disguise keeps the host's immune system from recognizing the pathogen. Although the body may still launch some nonspecific defenses against the pathogen, it will not produce more powerful targeted antibodies to attack it.

How Fungal and Protozoal Pathogens Evade Host Defenses

Many fungi release toxins that cause damage to host tissue and allow the fungus to spread its infection. Some also produce a capsule-like coating that works like bacterial capsules for avoiding phagocytosis. Other fungi can alter their metabolism enough to form resistance to antifungal drugs (drugs designed specifically to inhibit or kill fungi). Overall, however, fungi possess fewer evasive tactics than bacteria.

Microbe Basics

The species *E. coli* contains certain strains that are especially virulent in humans. These strains are called serotypes and differ by the substances they carry on the outside of their cells. The outer-surface substances help *E. coli* attach to host cells and evade certain host defenses.

Five different categories of E. coli's most virulent strains exist:

➤ Enterohemorrhagic *E. coli*: Releases toxins that damage tissue and cause bleeding

➤ Enteroaggregative *E. coli*: Causes persistent (lasting more than fourteen days), severe diarrhea

➤ Enteroinvasive *E. coli*: Secretes enzymes that help them invade tissue

➤ Enterotoxigenic *E. coli*: Causes toxin-induced damage

➤ Enteropathogenic *E coli*.: Causes diarrhea mainly in infants

Several dozen strains in each category exist. Each may have a different infectious dose. The most prevalent known to date to cause illness in people are *E. coli* O157:H7 and O104:H4, both enterohemorrhagic strains.

E. coli and other bacteria fit into subcategories based on specific carbohydrates that always appear on the outer surface of their cells. These carbohydrates belong to different antigen groups, identified by the letters A through T. Thus, *E. coli* O157:H7 always contains O antigen #157 and H antigen #7.

Protozoa rely mainly on two mechanisms for evading the host: by becoming parasites inside host cells or by antigenic variation. The *Plasmodium* species that causes malaria evades host immunity by entering liver cells and red blood cells. *Trypanosoma*, the cause of African sleeping sickness, produces a substance on its cell that the body identifies as an antigen, to which antibodies are made. But within a week or two in the bloodstream, *Trypanosoma* makes new surface substances, rendering the antibodies useless. As the body produces a new batch of antibodies, *Trypanosoma* changes yet again. The protozoan can make about 1,000 different antigens to constantly befuddle the host's antibody-production system.

Microbe Basics

A parasite is any organism that lives on or in a host usually at the expense of the host's health. Some parasites require a specific host. For example, viruses target a very narrow array of hosts consisting of no more than one to three species. Other parasites, like dog fleas, hop on any host they find.

How Viruses Evade Host Defenses

Viruses efficiently evade host defenses by existing only inside host cells. To destroy the virus would mean destroying oneself. Viruses further enhance their stealth in the body by frequently changing the substances on their outer surface, thereby making the body's antibody response less effective.

The hepatitis B virus invades liver cells. From this location, the virus releases a large number of "dummy" antigens into the bloodstream. As a result, the body feverishly produces antibodies to the various antigens even though these antigens do not harm the body. Once the body has reached full capacity for making useless antibodies, the actual virus begins its work of destroying the liver.

Viruses such as HIV infect T-cells that are required for normal functioning of the immune system. By this two-pronged approach to infection, HIV hides from phagocytes and other immune defenses and simultaneously weakens the body's overall immunity.

How Pathogens Cause Damage to the Body

If a pathogen could think, it might be saying at this point, "Okay, I've entered the host and escaped his defenses so far. Now I need to find a comfy place to grow." When pathogens settle down in a favorite type of tissue or organ, the real damage begins to the host.

Pathogens disrupt a body's normal metabolism by interfering with nutrient use, cell reproduction, or the structure and function of host cells. Pathogens do these things mainly through the action of enzymes and toxins.

Many bacteria, fungi, and protozoa use nutrients that the host also needs. The best-known nutrient-robbing activity is the siderophore. Some bacteria (*E. coli*, *Mycobacterium*) and fungi (*Aspergillus*, *Neurospora*) produce siderophores, which are compounds that tightly bind to iron. The siderophore holds onto iron tighter than the host's own iron-binding substances. As a result, a pathogen can absorb the iron it needs for survival while robbing the host of this essential nutrient.

Besides existing in host cells to avoid the host's defenses, some bacteria (*Streptococcus pneumoniae*, *Vibrio cholerae*) and all viruses have the ability to operate inside host cells as well. These are parasitic pathogens. In this scenario, the pathogen takes over the cell's normal reproduction. It does this by inserting part of its DNA into the host cell's DNA. This insertion ensures that every time a host cell reproduces, it also produces more of the pathogen.

Microbe Basics

The general structure of DNA is the same in microbes as in higher organisms such as humans. DNA's organization within a cell differs, however, between prokaryotes and eukaryotes. In prokaryotes, the DNA is a circular structure that is twisted into a dense coil called a supercoil. In eukaryotes, the DNA is organized around proteins called histones and folded in an exact way to help it fit inside the cell and make replication easier. Eukaryotes also protect DNA by storing it inside a membrane-bound area called the nucleus. Prokaryotes lack a nucleus and leave their DNA supercoil somewhat exposed in the watery contents of their cell.

Parasitic pathogens choose between two options inside the host. One option is to lyse (break apart) the host cell. This happens after a new generation of pathogens has been produced and the offspring are ready to enter the bloodstream. In the other option, the pathogen may take over much of the host cell's inner workings but allow it to stay alive. This process, called lysogeny, gives rise to generation upon generation of new pathogens. The host becomes a pathogen-manufacturing plant!

Some pathogens cause direct damage to host tissue by destroying it with enzymes or poisoning the tissue with toxins. The pathogen's enzymes help bring nutrients to the pathogen but at the expense of host cells. Toxins, meanwhile, are released from the pathogen and travel through the bloodstream and the lymph fluid to other parts of the body. The toxin weakens the host, enabling the pathogen to gain a better foothold in its temporary home. Although toxins can damage any part of a host's cell, about half of all known toxins damage cells by disrupting the cell's outer membrane.

Certain species of bacteria, fungi, protozoa, and algae produce toxins, or microbial poisons. The capacity of a pathogen to produce a toxin is called toxigenicity. Toxigenicity, therefore, makes up part of a pathogen's virulence.

Pathogens produce two types of toxins: exotoxins and endotoxins. Exotoxins are excreted from living pathogens and work in the host at places distant from the main infection. For example, an exotoxin made in the digestive tract during a food-borne illness can circulate in your blood and cause a headache. Endotoxins are part of the pathogen's cell and are released only after the pathogen dies and lyses. When either type of toxin enters the blood, the condition is called toxemia.

Both exotoxins and endotoxins give advantages to pathogens. Exotoxins allow the pathogen to weaken the host at a place different from the infection site. Endotoxins, by contrast, help the pathogen cause the maximum damage at the infection site, thus making the infection all the more difficult to stop.

Virulence

The first question that comes up when thinking about any pathogen is how virulent it is. Virulence determines the likelihood of infection and the severity of any disease from that initial infection.

Infectivity, invasiveness, pathogenic potential, toxigenicity, and infectious dose together determine a pathogen's virulence. The higher any of those factors are, except infectious dose, the higher the microbe's virulence will be. Highly virulent pathogens tend to have low infectious doses.

Many microbes have sections in their DNA called pathogenicity islands. These DNA segments contain genes responsible for virulence. Some of the most virulent pathogens have more than one pathogenicity island. In other words, these microbes are engineered to release the maximum amount of havoc on our health.

Target Tissues and Organs

Any progression from infection to disease can be summarized in these four steps:

> ➤ Encounter
> ➤ Entry
> ➤ Establishment
> ➤ Damage

Encounter between host and pathogen has to do with disease transmission, to be discussed later. Entry and establishment are the main components of infection. Damage to tissues and organs following the initial infection relates to the specific infectious disease caused by the pathogen.

Every pathogen of humans, animals, and plants attacks certain tissues or organs. Pathogens seek these special targets because of their unique set of virulence factors. Put another way, a pathogen finds a target tissue most compatible with its ability to infect, reproduce, and propagate a new generation of offspring pathogens.

Some pathogens do not need to penetrate into the body's deep tissues. On the body's surface or at an organ's surface, these microbes cause superficial conditions such as the following:

➤ Athlete's foot: caused by the *Trichophyton mentagrophytes* fungus

➤ Cholera: caused by a *Vibrio cholerae* bacterial infection of the small intestine

➤ Cystitis, bladder infection: caused by various bacteria

➤ Diphtheria: caused by a *Corynebacterium diphtheriae* bacterial infection of the upper respiratory tract

➤ Gonorrhea: caused by a *Neisseria gonorrhea* bacterial infection of the urethra

➤ Whooping cough: caused by a *Bordetella pertussis* bacterial infection of the upper and lower respiratory tracts

Other pathogens spread from the superficial infection site to tissues deeper in the body. For this reason, infectious diseases can be classified based on the target tissues and organs invaded by the pathogen:

➤ Skin

➤ Eyes

➤ Nervous system

➤ Respiratory system

➤ Cardiovascular system

➤ Lymphatic system

➤ Digestive system

➤ Urinary system

➤ Reproductive system

The worst infectious diseases attack more than one system at the same time. For example, in AIDS the immune system receives as much damage as the nervous system.

Skin and Eye Diseases

Pathogens that target the skin also include the species that infect the body through the mucous membranes. These pathogens tend to belong to bacteria, fungi, or viruses. Of the bacteria and fungi, they can be either frank or opportunistic pathogens. Some almost-microscopic parasites, such as mites and lice, also target the skin.

Common eye infections are caused by the bacteria *Haemophilus influenzae* (pinkeye), *Neisseria gonorrhea* (bacterial conjunctivitis), and *Chlamydia trachomatis* (inclusion conjunctivitis and trachoma). These bacterial infections are highly contagious and spread from person to person; trachoma is also spread by flies.

The virus herpes simplex type 1 causes the eye infection herpetic keratitis. Cytomegalovirus (CMV) is in the same virus family as herpes and causes CMV inclusion disease, especially in immunocompromised people such as AIDS patients.

The main protozoal infection of the eye is *Acanthamoeba* keratitis, caused by the microbe of the same name. This microbe encounters the host via water or by contaminating contact cleaning solutions.

Nervous System Diseases

Many pathogens or their toxins target the nervous system. This includes most of the known latent diseases, which hide in nerve tissue for decades before starting a disease. Following are the important bacterial diseases of the nervous system:

➤ Meningitis (*Neisseria meningitidis, Streptococcus pneumoniae*, or *Haemophilus influenzae*)

➤ Tetanus (*Clostridium tetani*)

➤ Botulism (*Clostridium botulinum*)

➤ Listeriosis (*Listeria monocytogenes*)

➤ Leprosy (*Mycobacterium leprae*)

Following are the important nerve-targeting viral diseases:

➤ AIDS (HIV): Poliomyelitis (poliovirus)

➤ Encephalitis (various arboviruses)

➤ Rabies (rabies virus)

The fungus *Cryptococcus neoformans* causes a type of meningitis called cryptococcosis. African sleeping sickness, caused by the protozoan *Trypanosoma brucei*, is a nerve disease as well. Prions also attack nerve tissue, illustrated by the human diseases Creutzfeldt-Jakob disease and kuru and the animal illnesses mad cow disease and scabies (sheep).

Respiratory System Diseases

The respiratory system is the target of numerous pathogens. Some pathogens infect mainly the upper tract and others target the lower tract. The most prevalent of all upper respiratory infections is the common cold, caused by several different rhinoviruses and coronaviruses. Other upper tract infections are caused by bacteria, such as the following:

➤ Strep throat (streptococcal pharyngitis): caused by various *Streptococcus* species, especially *S. pyogenes*

➤ Scarlet fever: caused by *Streptococcus pyogenes*

➤ Otitis media: caused by *Staphylococcus aureus* and various other bacteria

Bacteria, viruses, and fungi target the lower respiratory tract, where infections tend to be more serious:

➤ Tuberculosis: caused by *Mycobacterium tuberculosis* and *M. bovis*

➤ Various pneumonias: caused by the bacteria *Streptococcus pneumoniae*, *Mycoplasma pneumoniae*, *Haemophilus influenzae*, and *Chlamydia pneumoniae*, or the fungus *Pneumocystis jiroveci*

➤ Influenza: caused by the influenza virus

➤ Legionnaires' disease (legionellosis): caused by the bacterium *Legionella pneumophila*

➤ RSV disease: caused by respiratory syncytial virus (RSV)

➤ Histoplasmosis: caused by the fungus *Histoplasma capsulatum*

➤ Coccidioidomycosis: caused by the fungus *Coccidioides immitis*.

Cardiovascular and Lymphatic System Diseases

Like the respiratory system, the cardiovascular and lymphatic systems are a target of a vast array of pathogens. Mainly bacteria, viruses, and protozoa invade these systems. The following are cardiovascular and lymphatic system infections caused by bacteria:

➤ Gangrene: caused by *Clostridium perfringens*

➤ Lyme disease: caused by *Borrelia burgdorferi*

➤ Septic shock: caused by various bacteria, especially *Streptococcus*

➤ Pericarditis: caused by *Streptococcus pyogenes*

➤ Rheumatic fever: caused by *Streptococcus* in a group called Group A beta-hemolytic streptococci

➤ Anthrax: caused by *Bacillus anthracis*

➤ Brucellosis: caused by *Brucella* species

➤ Tularemia: caused by *Francisella tularensis*

➤ Ehrlichiosis: caused by *Ehrlichia* species

➤ Rocky Mountain spotted fever: caused by *Rickettsia rickettsii*

Of the many viral diseases of the cardiovascular and lymphatic systems, the following are the most well-known:

➤ Mononucleosis (Epstein-Barr virus)

➤ CMV infection (cytomegalovirus)

➤ Yellow fever (yellow fever virus)

➤ Hantavirus pulmonary syndrome (hantavirus)

➤ Dengue fever (dengue virus)

Protozoan diseases of the blood are less common in the United States than in other parts of the world. Most of the protozoan diseases in this country occur in immunocompromised people. Examples:

➤ Malaria (*Plasmodium* species)

➤ Toxoplasmosis (*Toxoplasma gondii*)

➤ Chagas' disease (*Trypanosoma cruzi*)

➤ Leishmaniasis (*Leishmania* species)

Digestive System Infections

Digestive system infections come almost exclusively from ingesting pathogen-contaminated food or water. Chapters 15 and 16 introduce you to the major pathogens of food and water, respectively.

Many of these pathogens, such as *E. coli*, appear in either food or water. In most instances of food-borne or waterborne infection, the bacteria, viruses, or protozoa came from fecal contamination, either from animals or from other humans. By contrast, fungal diseases of the digestive tract come from the ingestion of foods (usually grains) that have been contaminated by toxin-producing fungi.

Urinary and Reproductive System Diseases

Infections originating in the urinary or reproductive tract of men or women are often sexually transmitted diseases (STDs). Both systems are open to the external environment and both have the potential to come into direct contact with a person carrying a pathogen.

Like the skin, the urogenital tracts have their own normal flora that resists invasion by interlopers. Although urine is sterile, the urethra is home to a population of normal inhabitants, both bacteria and fungi. (As urine passes through the urethra, it picks up many of these microbes. Because of the extraneous microbes urine picks up, a urine sample given at a doctor's office is rarely sterile.)

Two factors influence the normal flora in the female genital tract: pH (the degree of acidity) and hormones. At birth and until a few weeks after birth, estrogens transferred from the mother's blood to a female infant cause glycogen to accumulate in cells lining the infant's vagina. Lactobacilli bacteria (also picked up from the mother) convert glycogen to lactic acid, making the environment more acidic (lowered pH). The acid serves to inhibit microbes other than lactobacilli for a while. Eventually, the estrogen effect subsides, pH rises, and other microbes increase in numbers to create the youngster's normal flora. At puberty, estrogen leads to another decrease in pH and the acidic conditions again cause a shift in the normal flora. Most adult women retain acidic conditions in the genital tract until menopause, when pH again turns neutral.

Many infections of the urogenital tract occur because of changes to the normal flora. A loss of the protective acidic conditions can alter the numbers and relative proportions of normal flora. Antibiotics, pregnancy, menopause, and some spermicides also alter the normal flora, which increase the potential for infection. The main opportunistic infection that occurs in these circumstances is candidiasis, caused by the yeast *Candida albicans*.

Urogenital infections occur mainly because a pathogen has been directly deposited on a mucous membrane. Almost all infections of the urinary tract are caused by bacteria, such as the following:

> ➤ Cystitis, inflammation of the bladder: caused mainly by *E. coli*
>
> ➤ Pyelonephritis, inflammation of the kidneys: caused mainly by *E. coli*
>
> ➤ Leptospirosis, disease of the kidneys and liver: caused by *Leptospira interrogans*, often caught by contact with infected animals

STDs occur in both men and women, many have no cure, and the incidences of some are increasing. To make matters worse, antibiotic resistance in STDs has become rampant. From 1988 to 1998, the incidences of antibiotic-resistant gonorrhea (ARG) doubled. In the following ten years, the resistance had increased about tenfold.

Gonorrhea rates have decreased slightly in recent years, but gonorrhea remains the second most common reportable disease. Gonorrhea infections are also a major cause of pelvic inflammatory disease (PID) in women. PID occurs when bacteria infect the uterus, cervix,

At the Doctor's Office

The CDC requires that certain diseases be reported by doctors to the centers and to the doctors' local public health agency. These are so-called reportable diseases. Reportable diseases are on the list because of their high threat to public health.

uterine tubes, and/or ovaries.

Untreated gonorrhea in males and females can lead to additional systemic infections (infections that spread to other body systems) such as the joints, heart, meninges, eyes, pharynx, and anus.

Following are the major STDs:

➤ Gonorrhea: caused by the bacterium *Neisseria gonorrhoeae*

➤ Syphilis: caused by the bacterium *Treponema pallidum*

➤ Genital herpes: caused by herpes simplex virus type 2

➤ AIDS (acquired immunodeficiency syndrome): caused by human immunodeficiency virus

➤ Genital warts: caused by papillomavirus

➤ Candidiasis: caused by the yeast *Candida albicans*

➤ Trichomoniasis: caused by the protozoan *Trichomonas vaginalis*

➤ Bacterial vaginosis: caused by various bacteria

Fighting STDs and the infections of other body systems requires diligence in personal hygiene, prevention of germ transmission, and adherence to any treatments prescribed by a doctor. Those treatments have been designed to fight particular pathogens at specific points in the pathogen's infection cycle. Thus, understanding the entire infection process is the best way to prevent and fight infectious diseases.

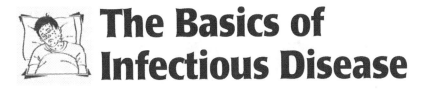

CHAPTER 4

The Basics of Infectious Disease

In This Chapter

➤ Learning about infectious disease by studying the infection chain

➤ The current status of infectious disease at home and globally

➤ Professionals who work on controlling infectious disease

➤ The main infectious diseases you'll likely get

➤ An overview of AIDS and the human immunodeficiency virus

In this chapter, I'll discuss our current knowledge of infectious disease. You will get an infection sometime in the future; you probably have already experienced many. This chapter points out why infectious disease is important to you, your community, and the world's population.

The best place to begin learning about how you get an infection and how it might turn into a disease is by learning about the infection chain.

The Infection Chain

By now, you probably realize that infection does not come from a single germ, lurking and waiting to pounce on any unsuspecting and otherwise healthy person. Microbes are by and large harmless; only a small percent cause infection in humans. There exist only about 250 pathogens known to cause disease in humans. Of those known pathogens, most do not cause fatal disease if a person's immunity puts up a reasonably strong fight against the infection and the pathogen's spread in the body.

Infectious disease, therefore, comes about only if a number of factors converge. The infectious disease cycle is sometimes also called the chain of infection. For infection to successfully move through a population, six interlocking links of the infection chain must be present:

> ➤ The infectious agent: Any bacteria, fungi, protozoa, or virus capable of infecting and causing disease in a susceptible host

> ➤ The reservoir (a constant source of the pathogen): A place in humans or other animals, or in inanimate objects such as soil, water, and surfaces, where an infectious agent thrives and reproduces

> ➤ Transmission to a host: Mode of transfer of the infectious agent to the susceptible host

> ➤ Entry into the host: Portal by which an infectious agent usually enters the host, including broken skin, mucous membranes, natural orifices, or artificial orifices

> ➤ The host's susceptibility: Factors due to weakened innate defenses, weakened immunity, or both that make a person less able to fight off infection

> ➤ An exit route from the host: Portal through which the infectious agent leaves a host to find another susceptible host

Microbe Basics

Contrary to what happens on television shows, a microbiologist (or doctor) cannot look into a microscope to instantly identify the next pathogen scourge. Bacteria appear as brownish-gray dots in a microscope. Microbiologists stain the cells with dyes to make them stand out from the gunk surrounding them. Even so, a microbiologist must study an unknown bacterium's favorite nutrients and other likes and dislikes before saying, "Eureka!"

Protozoa and fungi offer more clues to their identity because under a microscope they have certain distinctive features. Still, one look through a "scope" is not sufficient.

Viruses cannot be seen at all under a light microscope. They require advanced electron microscopes for viewing. Because of the distinctive shape of some viruses, images under an electron microscope are very helpful toward figuring out their identity.

Pathology is the study of the causes and outcomes of disease. In infectious disease study, pathology is concerned with each of the six links in the infection chain. Infectious disease cannot happen unless there is first a localized infection. Pathologists also study how disease progresses from a localized infection to other cells, tissues, or organs of the body.

The infection chain from the pathogen to the exit from a host is sometimes depicted as a straight chain, but it also can be a continuous chain. The continuous round chain reminds us that infectious disease stays in a host population for as long as the factors that sustain it remain.

Human society has been very cooperative toward pathogens. People live in dense populations, which helps germ transmission. People also do a remarkably good job of spreading germs to themselves and others. Sneezing, coughing, failing to wash hands, touching foods with contaminated hands, and sexual encounters are but a few of the ways humanity moves germs around. Humans have in fact ensured that germs never disappear.

Pathogens have evolved a few tricks of their own to keep from going extinct. The main tactic used by pathogens to ensure their longevity is to be sublethal. If all pathogens killed every person they infected, and killed swiftly, they would remove from Earth the very hosts they need for their survival. Pathogens must operate at a level of virulence that is strong enough to weaken a host, but not so virulent as to kill a host before the pathogen can reproduce and find a new host to infect.

Only one infectious agent, the smallpox virus, has been eradicated from the human population. Although a small number of government laboratories worldwide retain some smallpox viruses in stored form, the smallpox disease no longer exists. All other known pathogens have persisted to a greater or lesser degree, despite the best efforts of medicine to remove their reservoirs, block transmission, or treat the infected.

The Current Status of Infectious Disease

Why is preventing infectious disease so important? Because infectious disease is the leading cause of death worldwide. Cardiovascular disease not related to infection tops all causes of death globally, but all the different types of infectious diseases kill more together than does cardiovascular disease. Of these infections, respiratory infections do the most damage.

In low- and middle-income regions of the world, the major killers of adults and children are lung infections (pneumonias), diarrheal diseases, HIV/AIDS, tuberculosis, and malaria. The diarrheal diseases begin mainly from ingestion of contaminated water. Influenza and the common cold are also prevalent worldwide, and influenza in particular adds to the annual death total.

In high-income countries, infectious diseases are often not perceived as a major health threat. Although fewer lives are lost in rich countries compared to poor countries due to infectious disease, these diseases affect the overall vitality of developed nations by reducing productivity, resulting in lost work hours, and contributing to hospitalizations.

International health organizations cooperate when carrying out programs for stopping the spread of infection and treating people who have contracted an infectious agent. Groups like the World Health Organization (WHO) and CDC's National Center for Emerging and Zoonotic Infectious Diseases (NCEZID) set many of the standards that national public health agencies follow to block infection in their countries.

These groups work together and with other organizations to learn more about the following focus areas in infectious disease control:

> Emerging diseases: Diseases that are new or new to a certain region in the world

> Reemerging diseases: Diseases that were once thought to be under control and are now returning to the population

> Zoonotic diseases: Diseases of animals that can spread to humans

> High-consequence pathogens: Pathogens of high virulence that pose increased risks to the population

> Movement of infectious disease: Changing global patterns of disease incidence due to mass migrations of people

> Food-borne and waterborne diseases: Infections carried by food or water used for drinking or bathing

> Nosocomial infections: Infections associated with a stay in a hospital or similar healthcare facility

> Testing and diagnosis: Developing new technologies, such as polymerase chain reaction (PCR), for detecting pathogens in the environment or during an infection

> Surveillance and outbreak response: The measures taken by public health agencies to stop infection from spreading through a community

Academic researchers, medical researchers, epidemiologists, public health officials, and doctors work within each of these specialties. They focus on each link of the infection chain relative to the particular specialty. These experts also receive training on particular diseases or groups of diseases so that they can offer the most up-to-date knowledge and expertise to their peers.

Microbe Basics

Polymerase chain reaction (PCR) is a laboratory technique that was invented in 1983 and has revolutionized microbiology. This method permits a scientist to make millions of copies of a microbe's DNA from a tiny piece of DNA from that same microbe. With fewer than a dozen ingredients mixed together and a simple machine called a thermocycler, within a few hours the PCR process makes DNA quantities large enough to study further.

PCR has enabled microbiologists to track infectious agents through a community, identify the cause of a food-borne outbreak, and, most important, diagnose disease.

The People Who Work in Disease Control

Infectious disease control is an enormous industry. It involves a global effort at universities, companies, research institutes, and medical clinics. The doctor and nurse you first visit when sick with the flu or a nagging cold represent your first resource for information on what ails you. But these people are also at the end of a long line of information gathering so that you receive the best advice for care, treatment, and preventing future infections. Hundreds of people work behind the scenes for each strep throat diagnosed and each antibiotic pill dispensed. Meet some of them:

➤ Epidemiologist: Person who specializes in the factors affecting the frequency and spread of disease or other health-related events and their causes

➤ Pathologist: Medical doctor who studies the manner of spread, transmission, infection, and disease progression of pathogens

➤ Clinical microbiologist: Microbiologist specializing in the detection of pathogens in a sample from a sick patient and the identification of any pathogens in the sample

➤ Bacteriologist: Microbiologist who specializes in the study of bacteria

➤ Mycologist: Microbiologist who specializes in the study of fungi

➤ Protozoologist: Microbiologist who specializes in the study of protozoa

➤ Virologist: Microbiologist who specializes in the study of viruses

➤ Microscopist: Usually a microbiologist who improves the methods for viewing cells under a common light microscope or more complex electron microscopes

> ➤ Principal investigator: Person, usually a medical doctor, who runs a study on a new drug for treating or preventing infectious disease

> ➤ Bioengineer: Engineer who designs and tests new diagnostic equipment used in detecting infectious disease

> ➤ Statistician: Mathematician who collects and analyzes data for finding patterns within certain populations

The Major Infectious Diseases

The infectious diseases most familiar to you are the diseases that are most prevalent, either in your community or worldwide. Other infectious agents might be rare, but their consequences are so frightening, most people have heard of these agents. Some of these rare but deadly infectious agents are rabies, Ebola virus, anthrax, and Marburg virus.

Food-borne and waterborne infections are the most difficult to diagnose as to cause. These infections often go undetected or undiagnosed even after they have passed through a community. STDs also represent a special subgroup of diseases in which the mode of transmission is clearly defined. All other infectious diseases can be difficult to pin down in terms of the source, reservoir, mode of transmission, and spread through a population. The task becomes even more difficult when dealing with an emerging disease, because this type of disease is caused by an infectious agent that may never have been previously seen in the human population.

Common Cold

The common cold is by far the most common infection. In the United States alone, more than 1 billion colds occur each year.

Colds are caused by either rhinoviruses (about 70 percent of all colds), coronaviruses (about 30 percent), or a combination of both. Colds occur at any time of the year but may be a bit more prevalent in the winter or rainy season. The reason for the cold's seasonality may be due to people staying indoors more in bad weather, thus spreading germs more easily.

Cold viruses spread in tiny airborne droplets of moisture called bioaerosols. Sneezing, coughing, blowing your nose, or contaminating your hand with cold virus and then touching a face can be an effective way to spread the germ to others. In humid conditions, cold viruses can survive (retain the ability to infect) for twenty-four hours on inanimate surfaces.

Cold viruses attack the mucous membranes of deep nasal passages or the back of the throat near the adenoid area. They do not spread farther. Most viruses are deposited in the nose by fingertips and then gradually work their way back to the preferred infection site.

Fewer than thirty viruses are sufficient to infect. Like other viruses, a protein on the virus's outer surface binds to a substance on the outside of a mucosal cell in the nose. Each virus requires only eight to twelve hours to enter the mucosal cell, take control of the cell's replication process, and make thousands of new virus particles. The symptoms of a cold (runny nose, sneezing, watery eyes, nasal congestion, and possible headache, cough, and sore throat) begin about ten hours after the first new generation of viruses has emerged.

At the Doctor's Office

No drug has yet been invented to cure the common cold. Cold viruses come in hundreds of forms and mutate rapidly. No single drug could keep up with this ever-changing array of pathogens. Cold medicines are good for alleviating some of the worst symptoms of cold, including congestion, headache, and sneezing. Colds are the most common infection you will probably get in your life. Fortunately, they are not life threatening and even people with a weak immune system should recover from a cold without trouble.

Cold viruses infect a rather small portion of the body, but cold symptoms make a person feel like something much more serious is going on. The symptoms come from the body's reaction to the viruses in the mucous membranes. The body's first response involves the release of compounds that regulate the steps in inflammation at the infection site: histamines, kinins, prostaglandins, and interleukins. By doing what they are intended to do—dilate blood vessels, promote mucus secretion, activate sneeze reflexes, and stimulate pain nerve fibers—these immune factors make a cold sufferer feel utterly lousy.

Even if a person never develops all the classic cold symptoms—about 25 percent of cold sufferers do not—the body eliminates the virus in about three days to two weeks.

Because rhinoviruses have at least one hundred different combinations of substances that act like antigens on their surface, the body does not develop strong immunity against the next cold infection.

Lots of products lessen the severity of cold symptoms but no product currently approved by the Food and Drug Administration (FDA) cures or prevents the common cold.

Cold sufferers are most contagious in the first two to three days of cold symptoms. Fortunately, the telltale symptoms are easy to spot. To prevent colds, avoid others with obvious cold symptoms, stay rested and well nourished to keep immunity strong, wash hands frequently and especially before handling food, and avoid touching your nose and mouth.

Other tips for avoiding infection in cold and flu season are:

➤ Steer clear of restaurant salad bars

➤ Pass on free samples of cut fruits and vegetables at farmers markets

➤ Avoid bagels, donuts, and other handled foods at office meetings

➤ Decline to shake hands whenever possible, and if you must shake hands, keep your hands away from your face afterward

➤ Use alcohol hand cleaners when washing with soap and water is unavailable

Influenza (Flu)

Influenza in humans is caused by the influenza type A or type B viruses. (A third group, type C, causes much less serious disease.) The symptoms of cold and flu overlap and people sometimes have a hard time differentiating between a bad cold and a mild case of the flu. The flu's classic symptoms are fever, aching, headache, extreme tiredness, and a dry cough. The flu also has a greater chance of progressing into pneumonia and other deeper tissue infections.

The contagious pattern of the flu also differs from colds. Flu lasts longer than most colds. An infected person can spread infectious flu viruses a day before flu symptoms begin and continue to spread germs up to a week after symptoms first appear.

Another major feature of influenza relates to its reservoir. While humans serve as the reservoir for colds, each season's new influenza A strain begins in an animal reservoir, usually swine or birds, which also suffer from a form of the flu. The virus moves from animals to humans in a process called a species jump. This occurs in communities, often in Asia, where humans live in proximity to farm animals.

Each new season's flu virus may be the result of a mixture of the genetic material of two different flu strains. This blending of genes from two different strains creates a new strain in a process called antigenic shift. Antigenic shift makes it difficult for the body to mount an effective immune response against each seasonal flu.

Flu viruses spread in bioaerosols and can remain active on inanimate surfaces for three days or longer. The virus attaches to the mucous membranes in the throat and begins a localized infection there.

Tips for preventing the flu resemble those for fighting colds—proper hand washing, avoiding touching hands to the face, staying away from others who are obviously sick, and being careful when touching surfaces that have also been handled by others.

Unlike colds, vaccines exist for the seasonal flu. These vaccines may reduce the overall incidence of flu in a community but do not eliminate it.

Infections in History

One of history's worst flu epidemics began in 1918 at Fort Riley, Kansas, as soldiers returned home from World War I. Unlike most influenzas, this strain felled the young and healthy as readily as it attacked the elderly and others with weak immunity. Over two years, the 1918 flu spread worldwide, killing 22 million people.

In 2007, virologists studied tissue samples from people who had died of the 1918 flu. With today's techniques in analyzing genetic material, the researchers identified the 1918 flu as the H1N1 strain.

A very similar version of this strain reappeared in 2005 and again spread globally from its origin in Mexico. The current H1N1 is a mixed strain that started in birds and pigs. Its mixed genetic makeup worries epidemiologists who think the strain might be unusually adept at changing its conformation, making a flu shot against it very hard to achieve.

Lower Respiratory Infections and Pneumonias

Lower respiratory infections may include flu cases that have progressed into pneumonia, as well as tuberculosis (TB), acute bronchitis (*Bordetella pertussis*), severe acute respiratory syndrome (coronavirus), hantavirus pulmonary syndrome, histoplasmosis, respiratory syncytial virus infection, and chronic non-tuberculosis *Mycobacterium* disease (NTD). Many different bacteria cause pneumonia: *Bacillus*, *Chlamydia*, *Francisella*, *Legionella*, *Mycoplasma*, *Streptococcus*, and *Yersinia*. The main pneumonia-causing fungi are *Blastomyces*, *Coccidioides*, and *Histoplasma*.

Because various bacteria and viruses cause lower respiratory tract infections, the treatments for each differ. The best prevention, however, is standard: proper care of infected patients. This includes keeping an infected patient away from healthy people.

A half-century ago, sanatoriums for TB patients served as sites where the infected could weather TB and recuperate before returning home. This isolation—the most effective way to stop germ transmission—was viewed as a cruel sentence for getting sick and is no longer used. Today, TB has made a resurgence in densely populated cities. Dense populations are the places of highest risk for catching all respiratory infections.

Cures and preventions of lower respiratory infections have been hard to achieve. Antibiotic treatment of lower respiratory tract infections has been hurt by the emergence of antibiotic-resistant pathogens. In some parts of the world, TB patients have been infected with multidrug-resistant TB (MDR-TB), a strain that resists most of the classic TB drug treatments. MDR-TB is resistant to two of the main TB treatments: rifampicin and isoniazid. A newer strain, extensively drug-resistant TB (XDR-TB), resists these two drugs also.

> ### Infections and Disease
>
> The respiratory tract holds a large expanse of mucous membrane that serves as a common point of entry for various pathogens. The upper and lower tract, however, attract different pathogens.
>
> The upper respiratory tract consists of the nose, pharynx (throat), structures associated with them such as tonsils and sinus ducts, and the middle ear and auditory tubes. Colds, flu, strep throat, diphtheria, scarlet fever, and otitis media are the main infections of the upper respiratory tract.
>
> The lower respiratory tract consists of the larynx, trachea, bronchial tubes that lead into each lung, and the alveoli, which are small sacs that absorb air and make up lung tissue. Lower respiratory infections include pertussis (whooping cough), tuberculosis, and pneumonia.
>
> Bacteria, viruses, and airborne fungi are the main pathogens that cause these respiratory tract infections.

Vaccination programs have been partially successful. The best preventions against lower respiratory tract infections mirror those for cold and flu. Staying away from others who are sick, however antisocial it appears, remains the best preventive for any infectious agent carried in airborne bioaerosols.

Diarrheal Diseases

Diarrhea may be an unpleasant subject to discuss. As a result, this common ailment likely goes underreported. Diarrhea is the passage of three or more loose or liquid stools per day. Its main cause is pathogen-contaminated food and water. This includes water for drinking, bathing, and recreational waters (beaches, water amusement parks, spas, pools, etc.).

Various food-borne and waterborne bacteria, viruses, and protozoa cause three different diarrheas:

➤ Acute watery diarrhea, such as cholera, caused by the bacterium *Vibrio cholerae*

➤ Acute bloody diarrhea, such as amoebic dysentery, caused by the protozoan *Entamoeba histolytica*

➤ Persistent diarrhea, such as infections by the protozoan *Cryptosporidium*, that lasts more than fourteen days

Perhaps most of the foods associated with diarrhea outbreaks (raw fruits and vegetables)

carry pathogens that came from water contaminated with feces from either humans or animals. Thus, the best prevention against these infections involves watching what you put in your mouth. Chapters 15 and 16 examine the preventive measures you can take against food-borne and waterborne illness.

Infections and Disease

Diarrhea

Diarrhea is a hallmark symptom of many infections that enter the body through the intestinal lining. Severe diarrhea causes fluid loss from the body, leading to dehydration. This effect is life threatening to the elderly, young children, malnourished people, and those with already weakened immunity. Worldwide, diarrheal disease is a major killer of children under five years old, particularly in poor countries, where underlying health problems already exist. In a sad cycle of poor health, severe diarrhea causes the loss of nutrients in children who may already be malnourished.

HIV/AIDS

HIV jumped species from primates to humans in the 1930s, perhaps earlier. In the first decade of the epidemic that began in 1980, the presence of HIV in a person's bloodstream meant a certain diagnosis of AIDS, followed by death within one to a few years. An enormous cache of information has been accumulated since then on HIV's structure, mode of action, latency, replication, and treatment. Despite halting successes against HIV infection and AIDS, this disease remains a difficult challenge in global health. Remember, AIDS is primarily an STD, but it also can be transmitted by blood transfers in transfusions, accidental needle sticks, and intentional needle use by drug abusers.

The following is a list of the main features of HIV:

➤ It's a retrovirus, meaning it carries ribonucleic acid (RNA) as its genetic material and uses the host cell to convert the RNA to DNA.

➤ In the United States, infection is caused primarily by the strain HIV-1

➤ HIV-1 attacks T-cells of the immune system at a protein called CD4+ on the T-cell's surface.

➤ Untreated infection of the CD4+ T cells initiates various forms of the disease AIDS.

➤ The reduction of T-cells in the blood increases the chance of opportunistic infections by other viruses and bacteria, fungi, and protozoa.

➤ Diagnosis of infection is done by detecting anti-HIV antibodies in the blood.

The CDC has issued the following guidelines for defining the diagnosis of AIDS:

➤ Fewer than 200 CD4+ T-cells per milliliter of blood (compared with 1,000/mL in normal blood)

➤ CD4+ T-cells accounting for less than 14 percent of all lymphocytes

➤ One or more related diseases or opportunistic infections

➤ Increased incidence of anxiety, depression, dementia, and/or insomnia

Infections and Disease

The presence of AIDS-related diseases, or opportunistic infections, such as Kaposi's sarcoma, lymphoma, cervical cancer, encephalopathy, wasting disease, and psoriasis, help with the diagnosis of AIDS.

Following are the most common opportunistic infections associated with AIDS:

➤ Candidiasis

➤ Coccidioidomycosis

➤ Cryptosporidiosis

➤ Cytomegalovirus infection

➤ Herpes simplex infection

➤ Histoplasmosis

➤ *Mycobacterium* infections

➤ Toxoplasmosis

➤ Various pneumonias

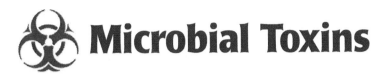 Microbial Toxins

In This Chapter

➤ Defining toxins and reviewing the different types

➤ Why toxins harm us and what we can do

➤ Important toxins made by bacteria, fungi, protozoa, and algae

In this chapter you'll become familiar with microbial toxins. Just as not all microbes in the world are pathogens, not all pathogens produce toxins. It's important to know a little bit about toxins because they act differently on your body than does a living microbial cell. The most important take-home message about toxins is this: Even after pathogens leave your body, their toxins might remain with you.

Toxins are poisons. Many different living things in nature produce them: plants, reptiles, fish, insects, and microbes. The most frequently encountered microbial toxins come from bacteria, fungi, protozoa, and algae.

What Is a Toxin?

A toxin is any substance that in very low concentrations acts as a poison in the body. A microbe capable of making a toxin is a toxigenic microbe, and this ability to produce the toxin is called toxigenicity.

Toxigenicity is one of several traits that make a pathogen virulent. Although some pathogens produce no toxins at all, the ability to produce toxins gives a pathogen advantages. For instance, toxins allow a pathogen to injure tissue without being present in the tissue. This remote-controlled type of effect helps the pathogen avoid an immune response by the body. Another advantage relates to the minuscule amount of toxin needed to cause maximum havoc in the body. From the perspective of a pathogen, toxins are very efficient.

Infection Vocabulary

Toxicity is the degree to which a toxin causes damage to tissues. A substance of high toxicity causes more damage than a substance of low toxicity. Toxicosis is the disease that results from the action of a toxin.

Another characteristic of toxins involves their composition. Almost all microbial toxins are made of either protein or lipopolysaccharide. This may not matter much to you when you have a toxin in your body and you feel awful, but it matters to the pathogen because different types of toxins behave in different ways.

Types of Toxins

Biologists like to classify things and then reclassify them! So just like there are various ways to classify infectious diseases, toxins can be categorized in a number of ways. A common way to group toxins is based on the tissues they target inside the body:

➤ Neurotoxins: Attack nerve tissue

➤ Enterotoxins: Attack intestinal mucosa (tissue lining the intestines)

➤ Hepatotoxins: Attack liver tissue

➤ Cytotoxins: Damage general tissues

➤ Hemolysins: Destroy cell membranes, causing cell contents to leak out

Another way to think of toxins is by the manner in which microbes secrete them. Some toxins are secreted from the microbe into its surroundings. These are exotoxins. Other toxins stay bound to the microbe and enter the surroundings only after the cell dies and breaks apart. These are endotoxins.

Exotoxins tend to be proteins and endotoxins tend to be lipopolysaccharides. This is an important distinction because for one, protein exotoxins can be destroyed by heating above about 175°F, thus, cooking can destroy them. Protein exotoxins also cause the body to produce antibodies against them. Antibodies that target toxins are called antitoxins. Antitoxins in the blood hold onto the toxin until macrophages arrive and digest the entire complex.

Infection Vocabulary

A protein is a large molecule made of carbon, hydrogen, oxygen, nitrogen, and usually sulfur. These components come courtesy of the main subunits of proteins, amino acids. Microbial, animal, and plant cells assemble proteins by stringing together specific amino acids in a set order. The final step in protein synthesis involves folding, twisting, or pleating the big molecule so that it can function as it should in the body.

All living things contain proteins that give the body structure—think muscle—plus specialized proteins called enzymes. Enzymes are proteins that regulate chemical reactions in cells.

The third point relates to endotoxins. Because they are lipopolysaccharide, they cling tightly to the membrane of the microbial cell. By removing pathogens when they're still alive, you remove the endotoxin. But by killing the pathogens in the body, a large amount of toxin pours into the bloodstream. In a classic case of damned if you do and damned if you don't, drugs that kill an infection might also release toxins into your blood. Toxins in the blood is called toxemia and it usually leads to the following symptoms:

➤ Exotoxins: Depending on the specific toxin, exotoxins cause diarrhea, paralysis, tissue death, and hemolysis

➤ Endotoxins: Cause fever, inflammation, diarrhea, intestinal hemorrhaging, abnormal blot clotting, and shock

Infection Vocabulary

Lipopolysaccharides (LPS) are molecules composed of polysaccharide and lipid. Polysaccharides are strings of eight or more simple sugars, such as glucose.

A lipid is a fatty molecule that does not mix well with water, like oil and vinegar. Also made of carbon, hydrogen, and oxygen, lipids found in nature are mainly triglycerides, sterols, and phospholipids. The latter is a molecule that has the element phosphorus attached to it.

Toxins Produced by Different Types of Pathogens

Toxins range from very dangerous to fairly benign, whether they come from bacteria, fungi, algae, and so on. To see what you're up against, it helps knowing the name of the pathogen that has caused your infection. Sometimes this detail doesn't come up in conversation with your doctor. Ask. The next time you are prescribed an antibiotic, ask the doctor, "What kind of infection do I have?"

Toxins from Bacteria

Toxins made by bacteria act either by doing direct damage to host tissue or by disrupting the normal actions of the immune system. Toxins have a particularly disruptive effect on cytokines, the proteins released by your immune system to help your overall response to infection.

Fortunately for us, some bacterial toxins need additional virulence factors in the pathogen to cause harm. For example, toxigenic strains of *Bacillus anthracis* cause anthrax disease only if the strain also produces a capsule.

Let's look more closely at the major bacterial exotoxins that affect human health: Shiga, botulinum, tetanus, cholera, and diphtheria.

At the Doctor's Office

When a person takes antibiotics to control a bacterial infection, the antibiotic kills the bacteria en masse or weakens them over a longer period. In either scenario, millions of bacterial cells release endotoxins into the bloodstream. Even though the bacteria may be gone, the effects of the endotoxins last a while longer. Taking antibiotics may therefore cause slight fever, lethargy, and other feelings of lousiness.

The following are some endotoxin producers:

➤ *Haemophilus influenzae*

➤ *Salmonella typhi* (typhoid)

➤ *Neisseria meningitidis* (meningococcal meningitis)

➤ *Staphylococcus* (ex. toxic shock syndrome)

➤ *Proteus* (urinary tract infections)

Shiga Toxin

The Shiga toxin is made by *Shigella dysenteriae*, a resident of human and primate intestines. Food or water contaminated by *S. dysenteriae* can result in the disease shigellosis, also called bacillary dysentery.

S. dysenteriae does all its damage to the intestines after a person has ingested it; it rarely ventures into the bloodstream. During infection, the bacteria enter the epithelial cells, which line the inner surface of the intestines. *Shigella* then multiplies inside these cells and spreads to adjacent cells, all the while avoiding the host's immune defenses.

During multiplication, *Shigella* begins excreting the Shiga toxin. The toxin damages the host by blocking protein synthesis. Without proteins, the epithelial cells rapidly die, leading to the hallmark symptoms of shigellosis: watery diarrhea with some blood, fever, abdominal cramping, and nausea. These symptoms begin about three days (range of one to seven days) after the host has been infected (the incubation period).

Methods to prevent various food-borne illnesses also prevent exposure to the Shiga toxin. This subject is covered in Chapter 15.

Infections and Disease

Toxins are dangerous because of the damage they cause at extremely low doses. The tetanus toxin requires only about 2 nanograms to cause illness. (A nanogram is one billionth of a gram. A gram is about the weight of a paper clip.) To put this in perspective, the Mojave rattlesnake is 10 times more toxic than any other rattlesnake. It needs about 12 mg to kill a human, or 12 million nanograms.

Botulinum Toxin

The botulinum toxin is made by *Clostridium botulinum*, which normally lives in soil. This microbe is an anaerobe (it cannot live if exposed to air) and produces endospores, rugged thick-walled forms that protect the bacteria against all means of destruction. Both these characteristics make *C. botulinum* a hazardous food-borne contaminant. The microbes live well inside the airless confines of canned foods and the endospore protects it from preservatives.

The botulinum neurotoxin causes botulism. In this disease, nerve cells (neurons) fail to properly communicate with muscle. The result is paralysis. The incubation period of botulism is eighteen to thirty-six hours (range of about six hours to ten days).

Botulism is a little trickier to prevent than other food-borne diseases. Most food-borne illnesses come from fecal contamination of the food, so paying attention to washing hands and proper cooking and refrigeration block many pathogens in their tracks. The botulism microbe, however, is in run-of-the-mill dirt, like that normally found on freshly picked fruit and vegetables. Improper home canning, home preserving, or manufacture of processed foods causes most cases of botulism.

Some tips greatly reduce your chances of botulism when doing home canning:

➤ Follow the standard recommendations for home-canning or home-preserving foods

➤ Follow food industry or government recommendations for food safety practices in the home

➤ Do not feed honey to infants younger than one year of age (a common cause of infant botulism)

➤ Discard all canned foods that are bulging

Bulging cans indicate that lots of gas production has taken place inside. This gas almost always comes from a microbe. And remember, because *C. botulinum* produces an exotoxin, the bacteria may be gone but the deadly toxin lingers.

Tetanus Toxin

The tetanus neurotoxin comes from another *Clostridium* species, *C. tetani*. This microbe also lives in soil but rarely ends up in food. The tetanus (also the name of the disease) toxin blocks nerve impulses to muscle and thus causes erratic uncontrollable muscle contractions. These spasmodic contractions usually affect the back, limb, and face muscles. The symptoms are stiffness in the neck and abdomen, arching of the back, difficulty swallowing, and, when affecting the face, lockjaw. Lockjaw is uncontrolled contraction of facial muscles.

The best prevention against tetanus is to keep wounds clean. Remove as much dirt as possible with soap and warm water, and flush with lots more water. Apply an antiseptic to the wound and cover with a bandage. The incubation period is two days to two months.

I often get questions from astute germophobes who wonder if covering a wound with a bandage might make conditions favorable for the growth of an anaerobe like *Clostridium*. Don't worry. Few bandages are airtight and they should be replaced with clean bandaging frequently.

Microbe Basics

The term *Shiga-like toxins* surfaces whenever virulent strains of *E. coli* cause food-borne illnesses. The dangerous enterohemorrhagic strains of *E. coli* produce this toxin, which is almost identical to *Shigella*'s toxin and behaves similarly in the body.

Cholera Toxin

This enterotoxin comes courtesy of the waterborne pathogen *Vibrio cholerae*. In the resulting disease called cholera, the toxin causes epithelial cells to release fluids and electrolytes. Watery diarrhea ensues, accompanied by nausea, vomiting, lethargy, abdominal cramps, and dry mucous membranes. Severe dehydration in cholera cases worldwide causes deaths each year. The incubation period is about two days (range of a few hours to five days).

Travelers to regions in Africa and Asia where cholera is prevalent must take extra precautions to seek safe drinking water and keep an eye out for foods that may have been cooked in or rinsed with contaminated water.

Diphtheriae Toxin

Corynebacterium diphtheria makes this cytotoxin, which affects the health of nerves, the heart, and the kidneys. Cell death in these organs is the symptom of the disease diphtheria. Diphtheria is transmitted by inhalation of contaminated bioaerosols from a sick person or by ingesting food or milk contaminated with *C. diphtheriae*. Many people carry low numbers of *C. diphtheriae* as part of their normal flora.

Septic Shock

Septic shock is a condition resulting from exposure to certain endotoxins made by bacteria. A shock is any life-threatening drop in blood pressure, and the word *septic* means that something bad has infiltrated the blood and the body's organs.

Endotoxins, like that made by *H. influenzae*, cause the immune system to overreact. Though substances released by the immune system provide critical defense against infection, too much of a good thing can be harmful. *H. influenzae*'s endotoxin prompts the body to release too much interleukin-1 and tumor necrosis factor (TNF). These substances in turn make blood vessels leaky. As you've learned, in normal infection fighting a slight increase in vessel leakiness helps fight infection. But too much leads to blood loss, a drop in blood pressure, and potential permanent damage to the kidneys, lungs, and digestive tract.

Septic shock is a serious illness and hits the elderly, the very young, and people with preexisting disease particularly hard. To make matters worse, antitoxins do not work as well in stopping endotoxins as they do against exotoxins.

Following are the main symptoms of this acute disease, in addition to low blood pressure:

> ➤ Rapid heart rate
> ➤ Heart palpitations
> ➤ Shortness of breath
> ➤ Cold extremities

Septic shock is a medical emergency. Patients require immediate treatment by a doctor and usually are admitted into the Intensive Care Unit.

Infections and Disease

Toxic Shock Syndrome

Toxic shock syndrome (TSS) is a serious illness caused by certain toxins classified as superantigens. Superantigens induce the sudden release of more than one type of immune cell as well as a massive amount of cytokines. A person with TSS experiences fever, vomiting, diarrhea, and loss of blood pressure.

Enterotoxins made by *Staphylococcus aureus* are the main cause of TSS. In menstruating women, TSS has been associated with the use of tampons. In these cases, the tampon provides a place for the bacteria to multiply to high numbers, with a resulting high output of the TSS toxin.

A related illness called streptococcal toxic shock-like syndrome (TSLS) results from exotoxins made by *Streptococcus pyogenes*. Both TSS and TSLS tend to affect skin and other soft tissues.

Mycotoxins: Toxins from Fungi

A mycotoxin is a toxin produced by mold or a mushroom. Mycotoxin poisoning occurs when people eat foods contaminated with mold or when people go wild mushroom hunting and return with a bag full of trouble.

Some of the most common foods to be contaminated with mold are grains. For this reason, mycotoxins threaten farm animals as much, if not more, than humans. Following are the main toxins from molds:

➤ Aflatoxins: Made mainly by *Aspergillus flavus* growing on rice, corn, sorghum, peanuts, soybeans, and cereal grains

➤ Citreoviridin: A yellow pigment and neurotoxin made by *Penicillium citreoviridae* mainly on rice

➤ Ergot alkaloids: Made by *Claviceps purpurea* growing on grains; affecting humans and farm animals

➤ Rubratoxins: Made by *Penicillium rubrum* growing on grains; causes hemorrhaging in animals and increases the toxicity of aflatoxins

➤ Slaframine: Made by *Rhizoctonia* growing on red clover; causes the disease slobbers in sheep and cattle

➤ Trichothecenes: Made by *Fusarium* growing mainly on wheat and rice

Tens of thousands of mushroom varieties exist—about five thousand in the United States—and to the uninitiated, many look identical. Despite the very small percentage of poisonous mushrooms among all species, each spring and summer brings new cases of mushroom poisoning.

Two important mushroom toxins are amanitin and phalloidin. Both are made by the mushroom *Amanita phalloides*, aptly nicknamed the death cap. Amanitin is one of many toxins classified as amatoxins, and phalloidin belongs to the phallotoxins. Amatoxins are more toxic and more likely to kill. The symptoms of both come on within six to twelve hours of ingestion of a death cap: abdominal cramps, vomiting, watery diarrhea, dehydration, and liver and kidney failure. The less toxic phallotoxins may cause swelling of the liver rather than complete organ shutdown.

Microbe Basics

A toxoid is a bacterial endotoxin that has been changed so it can no longer damage the body. Drug companies make toxoids out of dangerous toxins. A doctor then injects the toxoid drug into a patient to prompt the patient's immune system to make antibodies against the toxin. This type of drug is called a macromolecule (a big molecule!) or toxoid vaccine.

Aflatoxins

Aflatoxins produce the disease aflatoxicosis, perhaps the most common of all mycotoxin illnesses. *A. flavus* is the main culprit causing aflatoxicosis; a smaller number of cases are caused by *A. parasiticus*.

Aflatoxins withstand heating and affect a wide variety of animals. Operators of feedlots and poultry farms know that moldy grains or hay can have devastating effects on their animals because the mild heating that occurs in roughages cannot destroy the toxin.

Aflatoxins begin accumulating in grains in the field before harvest. After harvesting, prolonged periods of high humidity promote further growth of the mold. Of the numerous grains vulnerable to aflatoxin contamination, corn is the most common. Animals fed contaminated corn can secrete the aflatoxins in their milk and pass it on by that route as well.

People should avoid any grain or nut suspected of being stale or moldy. Food-processing companies have more than one process for detecting molds and throwing out moldy foods.

Infections in History

Beginning in 1692 in the area in and around Salem, Massachusetts, young girls suffered a mysterious illness. Their symptoms were seizures, convulsions, incomprehensible speech, trancelike behavior, and extreme sensitivity of the skin to touch. Times being what they were, the local clergymen swiftly diagnosed the root of the problem as witchcraft. The ensuing witch hunt and trials turned into one of history's darkest moments. Dozens of Salem's residents were accused of being witches, and many were hanged or starved in jail cells awaiting trial.

Researchers began delving into a possible medical cause for the Salem witch trials, which lasted only a few months before the townspeople returned to their good senses. They concluded that ergot poisoning could have been the cause of some of the odd behavior experienced in Salem.

An unusually damp spring and summer had preceded Salem's 1692 rye crop. The grain had been put up in storage for the winter and was used little by little. As the moist grain waited to be used, fungi grew throughout most of the harvest and excreted the toxin ergot. This toxin is now known to produce neurological symptoms, including hallucination, spasms, and hypersensitivity of the skin.

The fungus had long disappeared from history, but its effects will perhaps always be remembered.

Protozoal and Algal Toxins

Protozoa tend to live inside the digestive tract of animals and insects, or they are free-living in nature. Algae, by contrast, live in nature in freshwater and marine waters and on moist surfaces on land. Any moist surface that catches a few rays of sunshine is suitable for photosynthetic algae.

Each group has species of which little is known. (More than one microbiologist has remarked that more articles have been written on *E. coli* than all other microbes put together.) For example, a group of free-living microbes called dinoflagellates are often claimed by protozoologists to be protozoa whereas algologists claim them to be algae. One thing upon which biologists agree is the importance of dinoflagellates as toxin producers.

Dinoflagellates grow to massive concentrations in water. These overgrowths of microbial cells in the environment are called blooms. Blooms contain so many rapidly growing microbes that they suck all nutrients and oxygen out of water and cause fish and invertebrates to suffocate.

Blooms that go by the names of red tide and harmful algal blooms (HAB) produce high concentrations of toxins. These toxins have had injured marine mammal populations of the California coast and other marine habitats. The variety of known HAB toxins is listed below:

Brevetoxin: A neurotoxin made by *Karenia brevis* that causes massive fish kills; causes neurotoxic shellfish poisoning (NSP)

Ciguatoxin: A neurotoxin made by *Gambierdiscus toxicus*; causes ciguatera fish poisoning (CFP)

Domoic acid: Made by a species of *Pseudonitzschia*; causes gastrointestinal and neurological disorders, including short-term memory loss and disorientation; causes amnesic shellfish poisoning (ASP)

Infections and Disease

Domoic acid produced in large blooms of algae has harmed marine life populations along California's coast and other locations. Small invertebrates feed on the algae. These animals get consumed by fish and larger fish eat the smaller fish. Eventually, the domoic acid works its way up a food chain to large marine mammals such as seals and sea lions. The animals become disoriented and beach themselves. Unless rescuers react quickly to help the victims, some will die.

Domoic acid also affects sea birds that eat fish carrying the toxin. A massive poisoning of sea birds in 1961 along northern California's coast led to hundreds of birds displaying bizarre behavior on land. This event became the inspiration for Alfred Hitchcock's 1963 film *The Birds*. Microbiology goes to Hollywood!

Okadaic acid: Made by *Prorocentrum lima*; causes diarrhea in humans; causes diarrheic shellfish poisoning (DSP)

Saxitoxin: A neurotoxin made by *Alexandrium tamarense, Gymnodimium,* and others; infects snails, then poisons snail-eating fish; causes paralytic shellfish poisoning (PSP)

The dinoflagellate *Pfiesteria* also causes a neurologic illness in people exposed to infected fish. *Pfiesteria* was first discovered as the cause of fish kills along the Atlantic coast and tributaries in 1991. Decades later, this microbe remains a difficult study, mainly because it passes through about twenty-five different stages in a single life cycle. Scientists suspect a toxin at work in *Pfiesteria* poisoning, but the presence of one has never been shown.

PART TWO

Infection Transmission

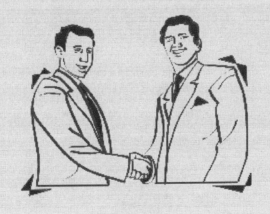

CHAPTER 6

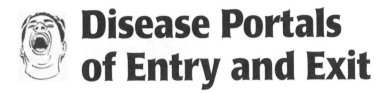 # Disease Portals of Entry and Exit

> ## In This Chapter
>
> ➤ Describing the body's portals of entry and exit
>
> ➤ Distinguishing natural from artificial portals of entry
>
> ➤ Learning tips on how to manage portals and stop germs from spreading

Portals of entry and portals of exit are the most overlooked aspects of infectious disease. Yet we would never get an infectious disease our entire lives if we were diligent in blocking all entryways into the body—portals of entry. And your family, coworkers, classmates, and community would have nothing to fear if we all were more careful about keeping our excretions—portals of exit—away from others.

Easy, right? Just stop sneezing without covering up, wash your hands before handling food, and don't cough directly on that guy in front of you in the theater. Of course, portal management, as I'll call it, also means dropping the habit of shaking hands, never picking up a baby, and never, ever being intimate with the person you love.

Most people do not want to give up all the experiences that come with human contact. We can still reduce the chances of getting infections and spreading them to others with good portal management.

In this chapter, you will learn the ins and outs of your body's portals.

Natural Portals of Entry

To cause disease, an infectious agent must accomplish the following four steps:

➤ Enter the host

➤ Attach to host tissue

➤ Evade the host's defenses

➤ Damage the host's tissues

Whether a pathogen causes disease by directly damaging host tissue or releasing a toxin to do the damage, any pathogen becomes completely harmless if it cannot get inside you.

Most pathogens have what microbiologists call a preferred portal of entry. These are the routes a pathogen prefers to use to enter the body. Some pathogens have only one route. The cold virus, for instance, uses only one route: it accesses you via the mucous membranes of the nasal passages. Cold viruses dumped on your scalp, knee, or even ingested will not create a cold.

Other more nefarious pathogens have a preferred portal of entry but can also use alternate portals. The anthrax pathogen, *Bacillus anthracis*, prefers to gain entry via the respiratory tract. But this pathogen can also enter the body through broken skin or the digestive tract.

Only two tissue types create our portals of entry: skin and mucous membranes. Skin is one of the largest organs of the body and offers the best protection of all our defenses against invasion by microbes. Mucous membranes form the lining of the respiratory, digestive, and genitourinary tracts, and the eyes and middle ear. Not as stout against invasion as skin, the mucous membranes serve as infection's main portal of entry.

Let's examine each portal of entry in more detail.

Skin

Skin is the outer covering of your body. As such, it is one of the main interfaces between you and your environment. Other than the eyes, ears, and nose, all senses come to you by way of the skin.

In a single day, thousands to millions of microbes come in contact with your skin. Most fall off or are washed off within a day or two. These temporary residents are called transient microbes. The permanent residents that cannot be removed by washing are your normal flora.

Except for the hair follicles and sweat gland ducts, the skin presents an almost impervious wall protecting your insides from the outside world. Even healthy skin can be infected, however. The main invaders of skin are certain fungi and parasites. An example of the latter is the hookworm larva, which burrows right through intact skin.

Fungi that digest part of the skin and thus cause infection are called dermatophytes. The resulting infections are cutaneous mycoses. Dermatophytes attack the skin by secreting an enzyme that breaks down skin's strong keratin proteins. Once they have weakened the skin, the fungi infiltrate the upper layers. Cutaneous mycoses have specific names depending on the part of the body they occur, all beginning with *tinea* for a surface fungal infection:

➤ Tinea barbae: Infection of the beard hair by various species of *Trichophyton*

➤ Tinea capitis: Infection of the scalp by *Trichophyton* or *Microsporum*

➤ Tinea corporis: Infection of the smooth, bare parts of the skin by *Trichophyton* or *Microsporum*

➤ Tinea cruris (jock itch): Infection of the groin by *Trichophyton rubrum* or *Epidermophyton*

➤ Tinea pedis (athlete's foot): Infection of the feet by *Trichophyton mentagrophytes*

➤ Tinea unguium: Infection of the nails by *Trichophyton* or *Epidermophyton floccosum*

Mycoses of the skin are difficult to prevent. The most effective approach involves keeping the skin clean and dry, wearing sandals in public shower or pool areas, and avoiding shared towels.

Infections and Disease

Many mycoses are not life-threatening but are nevertheless annoying. Superficial mycoses are infections of the outer surface of skin and hair, and they are examples of infections that are more of a cosmetic concern than a health concern.

In the United States, dandruff and tinea versicolor are the two main superficial mycoses. Tinea versicolor is the appearance of brownish-red scales on the trunk and possibly also on the face, neck, and arms. Both ailments are caused by the yeast *Malassezia furfur*.

Superficial mycoses become more common in the tropics, perhaps due to the humidity. Examples are black piedra, an infection by the fungus *Piedraia* that causes black bumps on scalp hairs, and white piedra, a *Trichosporon* yeast infection marked by light patches on the beard area.

The Respiratory Tract

A person inhales several thousand microbes each day, yet defenses in the respiratory tract help keep them from infecting the body. Any cold or flu sufferer can tell you that the system isn't foolproof.

The respiratory tract consists of the entire route from the nose to the lungs. Within this route, a microbe must slip past the nose hairs, the *ciliary escalator*, and phagocytes that work right in the mucus of the lower respiratory tract. Saliva occasionally flushes the inhaled microbes into the throat and to the stomach for destruction by stomach acids.

As a final one-two punch, coughing and sneezing expel plenty of foreign particles from the respiratory tract. Yet somehow, pathogens get through. Respiratory infections are among the most prevalent types of diseases seen worldwide each year.

Infection Vocabulary

This book refers often to mucous membranes because they play a critical role in protecting the body from infection, but they also offer pathogens a place to enter the body.

A mucous membrane is any sheet of cells that secretes the thick, sticky substance known as mucus. Mucus lubricates the mucous membrane-lined respiratory, digestive, and genitourinary tracts.

Mucous membranes belong to a category of body tissue called epithelial tissue. This tissue type consists of tightly packed cells that cover the outside of the body or line organs or cavities.

The term *mucosa* refers to an epithelial layer that lines the inside of an organ, such as the stomach mucosa.

The Digestive Tract

The mouth's saliva has digestive enzymes that should kill or inhibit most microbes. If microbes get past the mouth, they splash land in the gastric juices of the stomach. At a pH of around 2, few things should be expected to survive the stomach.

How in the world do all those food-borne pathogens get through our defenses and cause thousands of illnesses every year? Smallness counts for a lot during infection. Microbes hide inside pieces of chewed food on their way to the stomach. Although stomach acids degrade some of the food, the many small food particles that continue to the intestines hold millions of nooks and crannies that protect the microbes. Even microbes in water and other drinks can easily find bits of food in the mouth and stomach to shield them during their log flume ride to the intestines.

The intestines must look like paradise to a microbe. As long as the microbe can get by without oxygen—most food-borne pathogens can—the intestines offer everything else a microbe could ever want. There's plenty to eat, drink, comfortable temperatures, a perfect environment. Even the acids from the stomach get neutralized here and are no longer effective against microbes. In addition, the folds of the small and large intestines give microbes an expanse of mucous membranes larger than any other place in the body.

After the respiratory tract, the gastrointestinal tract acts as the major portal of entry for infection.

The Genitourinary Tract

Unlike the respiratory and digestive tracts, the inner sanctum of the kidneys, ureters, and bladder are normally sterile. Urine is sterile, too, until it picks up microbes as it passes through the urethra. Each organ also has unique characteristics that inhibit the growth of microbes. These main defenses are as follows:

➤ Urine's low pH inhibits many bacteria.

➤ Kidneys filter blood and produce urine, a process that makes conditions very unfavorable for microbial growth.

➤ Urination flushes the system several times a day, making it difficult for microbes to attach to the lining of the ureters or bladder.

➤ The vagina contains a large number of *Lactobacillus acidophilus* bacteria that produce acid and thus inhibit other microbes.

At the Doctor's Office

Few biological substances are as underrated as pus. This thick fluid is loaded with proteins, white blood cells (especially neutrophils), and cell debris made during inflammation. The accumulation of pus tells you that you have an infection and many cells of the immune system have rushed to the site to help kill it. Pus is a visible sign of an intense battle between your immune system and the pathogens.

Doctors examine samples of pus—actually, a clinical microbiologist does this in a laboratory—to determine the types of microbes present. This gives some indication of what microbe may have caused a superficial infection.

The color of pus also tells something about the infection. Normal pus is yellow. Reddish pus indicates the presence of blood and the possibility of infection deeper in the body. Blue pus (pus with a slight blue tint) indicates the presence of the bacterium *Pseudomonas aeruginosa*. This opportunistic pathogen is a common cause of hospital infections, urinary tract infections (UTIs), and, more serious, sepsis. Sepsis is the presence of a microbe throughout the blood and body organs.

Infections of the genitourinary tract are almost always STDs with the exception of opportunistic *Candida* infection. STDs also include the infections that enter by way of the mouth or rectum during sexual activity. More than thirty STDs are known and are caused by bacteria, viruses, or protozoa. Many microbiologists feel that STDs are out of control worldwide. These pathogens overcome the body's natural defenses for a number of reasons:

➤ High infectious doses

➤ Repeated exposure to the pathogen

➤ A preexisting or chronic disease that weakens immunity

➤ Antibiotic-resistant strains

Another factor contributes to the STD crisis: poor education concerning these diseases and how they spread. Many otherwise rational adults deny the STD problem in this and other countries. Parents often resist sex education in schools and this decision can delay getting information to those who need it most: teenagers who are becoming sexually active. The staggering amount of false and misleading information held by adults as well as teenagers regarding reproduction biology suggests that the STD pathogens have a bright future.

Some STD pathogens use alternate nonsexual portals of entry. For example, infected mothers can transmit HIV and hepatitis B and C to their infants. Hepatitis A, B, and C viruses are also transmitted through sexual contact. STDs also use various artificial portals of entry, which will be discussed later in this chapter.

Infections in History

Until about the 1960s, venereal disease (VD) was the name for sexually transmitted diseases (STDs). *Venereal* came from Venus, the Roman goddess of love.

Syphilis and gonorrhea have been in society since antiquity and had long been the only known VDs. For centuries, doctors thought they were caused by the same thing, although the exact pathogen remained unknown. In 1879, German dermatologist Albert Neisser discovered the bacterium that causes gonorrhea. It would be named after him: *Neisseria gonorrhoeae*. In 1905, the syphilis pathogen *Treponema* was first studied by German bacteriologists Fritz Schaudinn and Erich Hoffmann using a new generation of powerful light microscopes.

Treatment for these diseases did not appear until the introduction of penicillin in the 1940s. Eventually, other bacterial, viral, and protozoal infections were added to the list of VDs and the entire group of diseases given the more explicit name STD.

Eyes

The covering layer of the eyes represents an extension of the skin or mucous membrane. Many microbes infect the eyes, especially through the conjunctiva, which is a very thin mucous membrane that lines the eyelid and outer surface of the eyeball. The disease conjunctivitis is in fact an inflammation of the conjunctiva brought about by various infectious bacteria, viruses, and protozoa. This disease also goes by the names redeye and pinkeye.

Almost all types of conjunctivitis are extremely contagious, so beware of others showing the symptoms of reddened eyes, pus formation, and swelling of the eyelids. Transmission of the germs usually occurs when a person gets the infectious agent on their hands and then introduces the germ to their own healthy eyes, yet another example of why you must avoid touching your hands to your face.

Following are some important types of conjunctiva:

➤ Chlamydial conjunctivitis: Caused by the bacterium *Chlamydia trachomatis*

➤ Trachoma: A more serious *C. trachomatis* infection that permanently scars the cornea

➤ Neonatal gonorrheal ophthalmia: Caused by the bacterium *Neisseria gonorrhoeae*; infants become infected by the gonorrhea pathogen during birth

Keratitis is an inflammation of the cornea, caused mainly by a viral or a protozoal infection. The virus herpes simplex type 1 and the protozoan *Acanthamoeba* each can cause severe damage to the eye in these infections.

Ears

Many of the normal flora of the skin also live in the external ear canal (the auditory canal) without causing problems. If ear infections occur, they happen in the middle ear. The middle ear begins at the eardrum and extends a short distance to the inner ear, an organ that helps you maintain balance. The middle ear contains the eardrum and three tiny bones that help sense sound vibrations.

Infections of the middle ear are called otitis media. They occur when viruses or bacteria make their way behind the eardrum and begin multiplying there. These infectious agents often enter with water when swimming. Microbes that use this portal of entry are the respiratory syncytial virus (RSV) and the bacteria *Streptococcus pneumoniae* and *Haemophilus influenzae*.

In acute cases of otitis media, the sufferer experiences pain, fever, headache, and vomiting.

Infection Vocabulary

The disease otitis media is usually defined as an infection of the inner ear. Although few people will argue this definition, otitis is more accurately an inflammation of the ear.

When you see *-itis* at the end of a word, it means an inflammation. Thus, gastritis is an inflammation of the stomach lining, appendicitis is an inflammation of the appendix, hepatitis is an inflammation in the liver, and so on.

A word ending in *-osis* refers to a bad condition in the body. For example, mycosis is an infection by fungi and cryptosporidiosis is an infection with the protozoa-like microbe *Cryptosporidium*. (The suffix *-oses* is plural.) The *-osis* ending hasn't been saved exclusively for infections. Halitosis means bad breath.

Artificial Portals of Entry

The most common way to create an artificial portal of entry is to get a cut, scrape, burn, or any other kind of wound of the skin that destroys the near-impervious barrier to infection that skin provides. Think of all the ways you can damage the skin. Indeed, few of us make it much more than a week without bandaging the skin because of a cut or scratch.

The parenteral route of entry by an infectious agent refers to any access via the skin. In addition to the various types of cuts to skin, this portal of entry includes punctures, bites, splitting due to dryness, plus needle injections and surgical incisions.

Any microbe that can be carried into an open wound has the potential to cause infection. Therefore, no single group of pathogens prefers this portal of entry. You might think of the parenteral route as a portal of opportunity.

Preventing infection through the parenteral route will be discussed again when covering germ transmission and hygiene. Here are some quick tips for preventing infection through artificial portals of entry:

➤ Rinse all bleeding cuts, punctures, and bites with lots of clean, warm soapy water, and then apply an antiseptic followed by a sterile bandage.

➤ Seek immediate care from a doctor following any animal bite.

➤ Use an antiseptic on the skin before getting an injection.

➤ Surgeons and dentists should use only sterilized equipment in procedures that will break the skin.

➤ Don't become an intravenous drug abuser.

Portals of Exit

The happiest day for a person who has overcome an infection is the day all the pathogens leave the body. For pathogens, exiting the body of a host turns out to be a matter of survival of their species. A pathogen so deadly that it kills its host before it can move on to infect others will soon be extinct. Therefore, portals of exit are very important in germ transmission and critical in the life cycle of pathogens.

Pathogens tend to use a portal of exit that is related to how they entered the host. For example, the TB pathogen enters through the respiratory tract and exits that way. Food-borne pathogens go into the mouth, travel the length of the digestive tract, and pop out—you know where.

Epidemiologists, the people who study how disease moves through communities, take portals of exit very seriously. These portals are the means by which disease is disseminated in your family, church, school, workplace, or larger community. Although it may not appeal to you as a life's calling, there is value in studying the various ways that secretions, excretions, discharges, and tissues get around in society!

At the Doctor's Office

Sneezing and coughing are actions taken by the body to expel unwanted and irritating particles from the respiratory tract. Both actions are caused by involuntary muscle contraction in the upper respiratory tract. In a cough, the glottis (the sound-producing area behind the tongue) is partially closed, which helps accelerate the air being expelled.

Only one type of sneeze exists, although people vary quite a bit in volume and tone. Many different coughs occur, and doctors listen to their characteristics to diagnose bronchial, pulmonary, ear, and other infections, including the unique whooping cough.

For pathogens, sneezing and coughing is an effective way to get from one host to another. For instance, a bacterial cell measuring only .0001 of an inch in diameter can travel more than 6 feet in a cough and at least 60 feet in one sneeze.

Following are the main portals of exit and the substances associated with these exit routes:

➤ Nose and mouth: Saliva and mucus discharged by sneezing, coughing, talking, laughing, and kissing

➤ Anus: Feces as diarrhea or normal excretion

➤ Penis and vagina: Semen and vaginal excretions in STDs

➤ Urethra: Urine contaminated during bladder infection

➤ Eyes: Tears and other discharges

➤ Skin: Blood or drainage from wounds

Paying attention to portals of entry and exit is the best way to reduce your chances of getting colds and the flu, more serious respiratory infections, food-borne illnesses, and STDs. At the same time, you help keep your germs from spreading to others.

CHAPTER 7

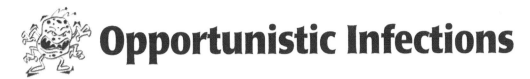 # Opportunistic Infections

---

In This Chapter

➤ Learning what makes an opportunistic infection

➤ The main microbes that cause opportunistic infections

➤ AIDS and the discovery of new opportunistic pathogens

In this chapter you will learn what opportunistic infections are and why managing them can greatly reduce the number of infections you'll get in your lifetime. For some lucky people, other than colds and an occasional bout of flu, most of their infections are of the opportunistic type. So keeping an extra vigilant eye out for them makes sense for better health.

An opportunistic infection is one caused by a microbe that is normally harmless. But there must be something more to it or all those harmless microbes in your surroundings would never infect. This chapter covers the circumstances that turn a benign microbe into a pathogen. It also introduces you to the opportunistic infections you'll most likely get at some point in your life.

What Causes Opportunistic Infections

Opportunistic infections occur for three main reasons. One reason relates to a host's susceptibility. People with a defective immune system cannot defend themselves against pathogens in the environment. Several conditions that put people at a high risk for infection were mentioned in Chapter 2. These conditions all increase the chance of getting an opportunistic infection, but certain health situations are known to further increase the risk of infection. These are the following:

➤ Immune suppression drugs for organ transplant patients

➤ Chemotherapy or radiation therapy in cancer patients

➤ Diabetes mellitus

➤ Cystic fibrosis

➤ AIDS

➤ Any other diseases that make the host immunocompromised

Infection Vocabulary

Immunodeficiency is a condition in which the body cannot make a sufficient defensive response when an antigen enters the body. Immunodeficiency may be genetic or can be acquired through a disease, malnutrition, multiple blood transfusions, or immune system suppressing drugs.

Being immunocompromised means that some part of your immune system does not carry out its normal function. An immunocompromised situation increases the risk of infection because the systems that keep away germs will eventually falter if exposed to a high dose of germs.

Another opportunity for infection occurs when a member of the body's normal flora grows beyond its typical numbers. Microbiologists know some of the factors that cause the normal flora to grow out of control, such as antibiotic treatment. Sometimes, however, the reasons are not understood and an innocuous resident of the body causes infection. Don't worry. In most cases, an opportunistic infection starts for a known reason: injury to the skin or mucous membranes.

A break in the skin barrier is a main reason for getting an opportunistic infection. If you get a minor cut, burn, or similar injury, you can reduce your chances of infection by tending to the wound quickly. On the other hand, some opportunistic infections occur without your control, such as an infection during a surgical procedure.

Consider what happens during abdominal surgery. A tiny puncture to the bowel can allow the escape of intestinal bacteria, such as *Bacteroides*. These microbes then enter tissue called the peritoneum that lines the abdominal cavity. The opportunistic infection is peritonitis. Surgeons are aware of the serious consequences of peritonitis and take appropriate precautions to prevent its occurrence. This is why surgery patients always receive treatment with antibiotics before and following surgery.

Infections and Disease

Primary infections are those caused by the first microbe that enters the body and establishes a colony. Infectious diseases are therefore characterized by the pathogen that causes a primary infection.

A secondary infection is caused by a microbe that enters the body after the primary infection has started. Some opportunistic infections are also secondary infections, for example, infections that follow an initial HIV infection in AIDS.

Meet the Main Opportunistic Pathogens

Certain microbes seem to be present time and again when opportunistic infections occur. A doctor might not always be able to tell which one of several microbes started the initial infection, but the recurrence of the following microbes makes it likely that each starts its share of opportunistic infections:

➤ *Pseudomonas aeruginosa*: This bacterial species is ubiquitous in water, including tap water, bottled water, and recreational waters such as lakes, pools, and spas. *P. aeruginosa* is also fairly common in moist soils. Its main opportunistic infections are pneumonia, UTIs, folliculitis, ear infections (swimmer's ear), and infections in burn injuries.

➤ *Candida albicans*: This yeast is a normal member of the flora of the skin, mouth, intestines, and vagina. It causes vaginal yeast infections in women taking antibiotics for a bacterial infection and can invade the blood in immunocompromised individuals, burn patients, and patients on intravenous lines.

➤ *Staphylococcus aureus*: This bacterium normally found in the nose and some areas of the skin participates in numerous secondary infections after another microbe has started an initial infection.

➤ Cytomegalovirus (CMV): This virus causes mononucleosis-type symptoms (fever, sore throat, swollen glands) in people with suppressed immunity, especially pregnant women and organ transplant patients. In AIDS patients and others with severely depressed immunity, CMV infects the eye's mucous membranes.

➤ *Pneumocystis jiroveci*: This protozoan used to be named *P. carinii*. It became a prevalent pathogen during the rise of the AIDS epidemic and is now known to cause life-threatening pneumonia in immunocompromised people.

➤ *Aspergillus*: Various species of this fungus live almost everywhere in the environment and can cause respiratory infections.

Microbe Basics

After *E. coli* and *Salmonella*, *Staphylococcus aureus* may be the most familiar microbe. This normal inhabitant of skin ends up almost everywhere in your surroundings because people touch their faces and other parts of their body, then deposit their *Staph aureus* on inanimate objects where others can pick it up. *Staph aureus* is very common in gyms, airplanes, offices, and any other place full of surfaces repeatedly touched by many different people. Poor food-handling techniques also make *Staph aureus* a common food-borne microbe.

The microbes listed above account for a large proportion of opportunistic infections, but many other microbes have the ability to behave similarly if they encounter a person with low resistance.

Symbionts

Symbionts are microbes that live with you and cause no harm, but they can harm others if they get loose and find a susceptible person. The most famous symbiont is *E. coli*, which occupies the intestines where it causes you no trouble. If you happen to ingest a large enough dose of someone else's *E. coli*, the situation becomes very unpleasant.

Following are other known symbionts:

➤ Echoviruses: A group of different viruses that cause intestinal infections

➤ *Streptococcus pneumoniae*: A bacterium that normally lives in the nose and throat but causes pneumonia in others

➤ *Neisseria meningitidis*: A bacterium of the respiratory tract that causes meningitis in others.

Microbe Basics

Showering is important to good hygiene. It removes dirt, dead skin cells, excess sebum and sweat, and various microbes. The normal flora of your skin attaches tightly to skin cells and the majority do not get washed away in the shower. By contrast, the microbes you pick up on your hands or by touching a microbe-laden object (or another person) are transient microbes. These microbes have not had a chance to form a strong attachment to skin. As a result, a shower removes most of these transient microbes, some of which could be pathogenic.

The normal flora that lives in peace with you also protects you by repelling many frank pathogens. But the medical profession has justifiable worries over the expanding list of microbes that now resist more than one antibiotic. Could a population of antibiotic-resistant species dwell within your normal flora? Antibiotic use destroys some of the normal flora. Undoubtedly, some of the survivors stay alive because they have features that make them more resistant to antibiotics than other microbes. This is the first step in developing a brand new strain that resists antibiotics.

Infections and Disease

Sick building syndrome (SBS) is a situation in which an excess of irritants inside a building affect the health of the people who spend time inside that building. The irritations may be either chemicals or microbes. The main microbes associated with SBS are the molds *Aspergillus*, *Penicillium*, *Mucor*, *Cladosporium*, and *Stachybotrys*. These fungi contact the skin and their spores irritate the mucous membranes of the respiratory tract.

The exact causes of SBS are unknown and this condition remains controversial because some people doubt it is real. The perceptions of people suffering from SBS are admittedly hard to diagnose. Workers who spend lots of time inside buildings with sealed windows, near-airtight doors, and an internal climate control system tend to report symptoms of SBS. These symptoms are headache, fatigue, difficulty concentrating, and various irritations of the skin.

AIDS and Opportunistic Infection

Nothing in medical history brought home the message of opportunistic infections more than the AIDS epidemic that began in the 1980s. In the early history of the epidemic, doctors felt helpless in fighting an unknown pathogen as well as a series of infections that seemed unrelated, yet were causing a mounting death toll. Those infections we now know were opportunistic and were the result of the drop in immune cells in people infected with HIV.

When HIV invades the immune system's CD4 T-cells, the body loses a major defense against other infectious agents. As the AIDS epidemic continued unabated for a decade, hospitals saw an alarming rise in secondary infections in their patients. The main opportunistic infections of people infected with HIV, but untreated for it, were the following:

> ➤ *Candida* infections: Often the first infections to appear about five years after the initial HIV infection.

> ➤ Tuberculosis: TB rates rose in HIV-positive individuals about six years after the initial HIV infection.

> ➤ *Pneumocystis* pneumonia: This normally rare disease showed up in high incidence in HIV-positive people seven to nine years after HIV exposure.

> ➤ *Cryptococcus neoformans*: This fungal infection often accompanied pneumonia.

> ➤ Cytomegalovirus infections: Eye infections showed up in abnormally high incidence in AIDS patients.

You might now realize that some opportunistic infections are preventable while others might be out of your control. The prevalence of antibiotic-resistant microbes in our environment offers no comfort, either. Fortunately, most opportunistic infections are of the manageable kind that occurs at the skin. Watch those skin injuries. Wash them, treat them with antiseptics or at least soap and water, and have deep injuries and bites checked immediately by a doctor.

CHAPTER 8

Epidemiology and the Basics of Disease Transmission

In This Chapter

➤ The basics of epidemiology science and its terms

➤ Learning the difference between outbreaks and epidemics

➤ Learning the types of epidemics and how to spot them

➤ Distinguishing between disease prevalence and frequency

➤ What to do during an epidemic

In this chapter you will be introduced to one of the most important aspects of infection, its transmission. To introduce you to transmission, this chapter begins first with the science called epidemiology. Epidemiologists spend significant time studying how disease is transmitted through communities.

If you learn nothing else about infection, learn the basics of transmission. By learning how to block disease transmission, you will greatly reduce your chance of infection.

An Introduction to Epidemiology

Epidemiology is the science of when and where diseases occur and how they move through populations. Epidemiologists study the patterns of how infectious diseases enter communities, but they also study the occurrences of accidents, poisonings, suicides, environmental hazards (air pollution, toxic chemical exposure, radiation, etc.), and health-related occurrences associated with disasters. As an example, it was epidemiologists who discovered the effects of chemical exposure following the 2001 World Trade Center collapse and the infections that surfaced in the Gulf region after Hurricane Katrina.

Infections in History

Modern epidemiology began in the mid-1800s in London during repeated waterborne cholera outbreaks. Rather than throw up his hands in frustration as others seemed to be doing, physician John Snow led an investigation into the cause of a particular series of outbreaks in Soho.

By taking on the tedious task of gathering information from households and taverns in the neighborhood with a high incidence of cholera, Snow determined that almost all had used a public water pump located on Broad Street. To test his theory, Snow had the pump's handle removed. New cases of cholera began to drop almost at once. (Snow also surmised that the infectious agent was multiplying in the city's water. In this way he came close to discovering the cholera pathogen, which would not be discovered for another fifty years.)

By these simple actions, Snow and his team invented epidemiology, the surveillance, investigation, and control of disease.

Epidemiologists gather as much information on potential hosts of infection as they collect on pathogens. Some illnesses occur because a pathogen has infiltrated society at a particular physical location. For example, good epidemiological work can pinpoint an outbreak of food-borne illness to a certain part of town, a specific restaurant, a particular dish on the menu, and the contaminated ingredient.

A few words about terms used in disease transmission are in order. The news media use these terms frequently, so let's be clear on the distinctions:

➤ Outbreak: The sudden unexpected occurrence of an infection or disease in a given population. Outbreaks usually occur in small populations such as dormitories, campuses, or towns.

➤ Epidemic: A disease that quickly increases above normal levels in a large population. Epidemics usually occur in large populations such as found in a city, region, or country.

➤ Endemic: A disease that is constantly present in a given population, usually at a steady low frequency.

➤ Pandemic: An epidemic that has spread across several continents.

The Role of Epidemiologists

For some diseases, epidemiologists must connect the dots between disease and a particular type of host. Thus, epidemiologists collect as much data as they can on age, sex, occupation, personal habits, workplace, socioeconomic status, immunization history, and family health history. All these factors help explain why infection strikes certain people and not others.

Finally, epidemiologists suggest the best ways to block transmission of a pathogen once it and its source have been identified. To achieve their goals, epidemiologists take part in the following practices related to community health:

➤ Immunization programs

➤ Water treatment

➤ Sewage treatment and disposal

➤ Community sanitation programs and trash pickup

➤ Animal- and insect-control programs

➤ Farm animal husbandry and health practices

➤ Food processing, transporting, and inspecting

➤ Screening of blood and tissues used in health care

➤ Improved nutrition programs for building immunity

Infection Vocabulary

Mortality rate is a measure of how deadly a disease is in a population. Mortality equals the number of deaths due to a given disease divided by the total number of people infected with the disease.

Morbidity rate is a measure of how many people develop a given disease in a population during a specific time period. Morbidity equals the number of new cases of the disease divided by the number of susceptible people in a population. Morbidity rate is therefore similar to incidence.

For the same disease, morbidity rate should always be higher than the mortality rate. The closer these two values become, the more deadly the disease.

Epidemiologists play a vital role in helping maintain overall health in a community and in the nation.

Types of Epidemiology

The broad subject of epidemiology has been divided into three main specialties: descriptive, analytical, and experimental.

Descriptive epidemiology is concerned with collecting data at the time of a disease outbreak. This specialty helps health officials figure out when an outbreak occurred, where it started, and the most likely source of the pathogen.

With analytical epidemiology, an epidemiologist looks at the history of a community before an outbreak occurred. The purpose here is to find reasons for the outbreak, especially why some people got sick and others did not.

Epidemiologists who specialize in experimental epidemiology test a theory on disease in a segment of the population. The easiest example is drug testing. The scientists might divide a group of infected people into groups. One group gets a drug known to kill pathogen A and the other group gets a placebo. If pathogen A begins to disappear from the group receiving the drug, the scientists know they have a pretty good idea that pathogen A started the outbreak. Experiments like this need two groups, drug versus placebo, so the scientists can compare the variety of signs and symptoms that might appear in all people.

Signs of an Epidemic

Case reporting is a procedure used by doctors and other healthcare workers to keep track of disease outbreaks. When a certain infection or disease has been diagnosed in a patient, the health professional reports it to local and national health agencies. These agencies compile the information and alert doctors' offices and the public that an outbreak is in progress. (The world is not a perfect place. Often the information gets to all these offices after the outbreak has already ended.)

Case reporting is thus an important first step in spotting a new outbreak or an epidemic. Conversely, if a disease goes unreported, then health care professionals and the public will have a harder time controlling it. You can't fight an enemy if you don't know it exists. Unfortunately, not every infectious disease is reportable, that is, doctors must notify health agencies as soon as they see it in a patient. Only about seventy-five infectious diseases are reportable to our national health agency, the CDC. The CDC lists on its website the current lineup of reportable diseases; search "nationally notifiable infectious conditions."

What about all the infections that do not need to be reported to health agencies? For instance, some food-borne illnesses require a report (botulism, *E. coli*, *Salmonella*, *Shigella*, and *Listeria*), but many others do not. Epidemiologists can be clever in figuring out if a community has an ongoing outbreak of a non-reportable pathogen. Following are some of the clues that have been used for spotting outbreaks:

➤ Increased sales of cold and cough medicine

➤ Increased requests at pharmacies for medicines to sooth a sore throat, fever, or diarrhea

➤ Increased sales of facial tissue and toilet paper

➤ High absenteeism in schools or workplaces

Any sudden increase in appointments at doctors' offices also is viewed as a warning that something bad may be spreading through a community.

Prevalence, Incidence, and Frequency

Epidemiologists use statistics to monitor the many cases of various diseases reported to health agencies. Some diseases, such as anthrax, occur in the United States at a low frequency. Others, such as food-borne illnesses, show up often and in many people. Epidemiologists therefore use two terms in their statistics: prevalence and frequency.

Prevalence is the number of people in a population with a given infection at any particular time. Scientists don't care when a person first contracted the infection when calculating prevalence. That is, people who have had a given infection for two years or two weeks are both included when calculating prevalence.

Incidence is almost like prevalence. It is the number of people in a population that first get the infection at a particular time. In other words, epidemiologists tally up the new cases of infection A diagnosed during a specific week to calculate incidence.

Scientists usually express prevalence and incidence as a percent. For example, the prevalence of infection B in Metropolis City is 10 percent.

For the mathematically inclined, prevalence equals the number of people with the disease divided by the total number of people in the population. Incidence equals the number of people who newly develop the disease during a set time period divided by the total number of people.

To keep everything in standard terms from one population to the next, epidemiologists like to report prevalence and incidence as the number of cases per 100,000 people. This eliminates any discrepancy when comparing big Metropolis City to tiny Podunk Village.

Both prevalence and incidence are ways of expressing the frequency in which a disease occurs in a population. By working with frequency rather than absolute numbers of cases, epidemiologists get an idea of whether a disease is increasing, decreasing, or staying the same in a population.

Infections in History

Florence Nightingale was a British nurse serving military troops during the Crimean War. Among her nonstop duties of tending the injured, cooking, and cleaning uniforms, Nightingale kept detailed notes on the medical conditions of the battlefield. In 1858, she published a 1,000-page report on her observations of food quality, infection, and disease. In it, she made several recommendations on how to improve on the squalid, unsanitary conditions in medical tents and military hospitals.

Nightingale's writings and opinions helped reform medical care for the military and the nursing profession, and promoted women's rights. In large part because of her detailed recordkeeping, Nightingale became the first female admitted to the Statistical Society. Her insight on society in general, and military medical care in particular, made her a legend.

Infectious Disease Transmission

Chapters 10, 11, and 12 give details on specific aspects in disease transmission. Let's take a big picture view of transmission as it relates to community health.

Pathogens spread through a community using different modes of travel called methods of transmission, which include the following:

➤ Airborne: The spread of germs inside tiny moisture droplets called bioaerosols

➤ Contact: Getting a germ by touching a living organism that carries it

➤ Vehicle: Getting a germ by touching a nonliving (inanimate) object that carries it

➤ Vector: The spread of germs by insects or animals

What You Should Do During an Epidemic

It may seem hard enough to avoid infection on your best day. What should you do then when an epidemic strikes? The odds are greater you'll get sick, but you may feel helpless to stop infection when everyone else around you seems to be sick.

We have demands in the workplace and at school, and we have responsibilities at home. How often have you heard someone say, "I don't have time to be sick"? You may have said this yourself. When we ignore the signals our bodies are giving us—sneezing, coughing, sore throat, chills, upset stomach—we perpetuate disease. Ignoring the clues of infection helps small outbreaks turn into large epidemics.

What if you are stuck right in the middle of an epidemic? Would you know how to avoid getting sick without sealing yourself into a cocoon and staying there for a week, maybe more? Here are some things to do in the case of a flu epidemic. Some of these actions are altruistic and will benefit your community. Other actions are purely selfish but are intended to keep you well when everyone else is "dropping like flies."

Following are actions you should take during a flu epidemic to avoid getting sick:

➤ Report your symptoms to a doctor or a pharmacist: Don't feel silly for speaking up. Most infections turn into outbreaks and outbreaks turn into epidemics because critical information on prevention got to the proper authorities too late.

➤ Stay home: This means don't go to work, school, the gym, the mall, the grocery store, etc. Within reason, avoiding crowds of germ-carrying people stops the germ from spreading. It's not an easy one to accomplish, but enough technology now exists for telecommuting, shopping online, and having purchases delivered to your door so that avoiding germs is possible.

➤ Stop sharing: Towels, sheets, utensils, toothbrushes, food, lip balm, and a variety of inanimate objects carry germs. At home, a sick family member should have his or her own stuff to contaminate as needed. Keep the uncontaminated items for the healthy members of the household.

➤ Be a healthy, useful employee rather than a sick, useless one: There's a reason for the phrase "calling in sick." Unfortunately, many companies value employees who drag themselves into the workplace when sick and frown on those who stay home. If you must go into work, avoid the doughnut cart, the cafeteria, and the lunch truck. Avoid also using another person's keyboard, mouse, pens, and phone. Clean shared equipment with an alcohol or disinfectant wipe before using them. The list of shared items seems endless, but think about the buttons on the copier, printer, fax machine, microwave, vending machine, elevator, and audio/visual equipment. Avoid water fountains. Avoid everything; you get the idea.

➤ Use disinfectants: If you prefer not to use chemicals around your home and work, an epidemic is an appropriate time to break this tradition. Using a disinfectant according to the directions on the container has been proven to lower the number of germs and block transmission.

➤ Follow doctor's orders: People follow doctor's orders to stay home, rest, and eat well until they feel better. Feeling better is subjective, however, and spreading germs still happens even after the worst of the symptoms have passed.

➤ Be antisocial: Remember that a portion of a population will be asymptomatic carriers of a germ. That is, these people spread infection but they never get sick. The answer is to become a little more antisocial during an epidemic. Decline dinner or movie invitations, avoid shaking hands, and run like the devil if you see someone sneezing all over the place!

Knowing the Pattern of Disease

Epidemics slow when the proportion of resistant people is larger than the susceptible ones in a population. An infectious disease rolls through a population like a wave. Though some waves are tall and swift, others are shorter and more gradual. The tall, fast wave might be indicative of an acute illness. The more gradual wave might indicate a chronic illness. Either type of wave still means an infection is sweeping through the population. It helps to know the patterns of a disease so that you understand your body's process and you understand what others may be going through.

Infection Vocabulary

An acute disease is sharp and severe, has a rapid onset measured in hours (not more than a couple days), gives severe symptoms, and then goes away quickly. The flu is an acute disease.

A chronic disease takes a long time after the initial infection to produce symptoms and lasts for a long time, measured in weeks or years. Sometimes chronic diseases show little change over periods of several months. Chronic diseases also leave the body slowly. TB is a chronic disease.

Any disease passes through stages as it develops and then subsides in your body. In fast-moving epidemics, most people might be experiencing the same stage at roughly the same time. In epidemics that develop more slowly, people in the same population might be at various stages of disease. In this case, you must remember that everyone is a potential germ carrier.

Here are the stages of an infectious disease:

➤ Incubation period: The time interval between the initial infection by the pathogen and the start of disease symptoms

➤ Prodromal period: A short period following incubation in which symptoms such as headache or general body ache indicate an infection may be present

➤ Illness period: The period when you know you are sick and experience symptoms characteristic of the disease. Highly virulent pathogens might cause the person to die during this period.

➤ Decline period: This means the decline of the pathogen, not the patient! During this time, symptoms lessen but the body's resistance to infection remains low. Secondary infections can occur during the decline period.

➤ Convalescence period: The period of time required for the body to regain full strength and return to its healthy state.

Infections and Disease

Disease carriers play an integral part in keeping a disease active in a population. A carrier is an infected person who acts as a source of infection in others.

Several types of carriers exist:

➤ Active carrier: Easiest to spot, this person has an obvious illness.

➤ Healthy carrier: The opposite of an active carrier in terms of knowing who to avoid. Healthy carriers display no outward signs of illness but can nevertheless spread infection.

➤ Incubatory carrier: One who is incubating the pathogen in large numbers but who is not yet sick.

➤ Convalescent carrier: One who has recovered from the worst of the illness but continues to harbor large numbers of the pathogen.

Remember also that carriers may be grouped as symptomatic and asymptomatic. The former shows outward signs of illness and the latter does not. Some people, like Typhoid Mary, can live their entire life as an asymptomatic carrier yet spread sickness far and wide.

The easiest disease stage to notice in others and you is the illness period when symptoms are raging. Remember, however, that several diseases are also contagious during the incubation period and the convalescence period. The flu and colds can be transmitted during incubation as can hepatitis B, measles, AIDS, typhoid, and gonorrhea. Diseases that remain transmissible during convalescence are typhoid, cholera, and *pneumococcal pneumonia*.

Infections in History

Some epidemics are on the rise in certain parts of the world. Certain STDs offer an example. In general, however, medical care improves each year. When, then, do epidemics disappear? Why do new diseases emerge or ones we thought were controlled remerge?

Too many changing factors in society exist for a scholar to name one reason for the potential rise in epidemics. Following are some of the factors that help sustain epidemics or turn them into pandemics:

➤ Prevalence of global travel

➤ Political conflicts that displace large numbers of people

➤ Rising poverty that leads to poor sanitation and malnutrition

➤ Large-scale food processing and distribution

➤ Climate changes that affects the breeding of insect and animal vectors

Symptoms seem to be nature's way of warning you of the potential for infection. But even with all the sneezing and coughing going on, microbes remain invisible. That is why fighting infection is at least a two-step process. The first step is to avoid someone with clear signs of disease, the second is to think about germ transmission even though you cannot see the germs around you.

CHAPTER 9

 # Outbreaks and Epidemics

In This Chapter

➤ The features of infection outbreaks and epidemics

➤ How outbreaks turn into epidemics

➤ The role of reservoirs in epidemics

➤ Types of epidemics and the current important epidemics

➤ Details on influenza and the AIDS epidemics

In this chapter you will learn about specific types of outbreaks and epidemics. The chapter focuses on the main types of infections most likely to affect you, your family, or your community at some point in your life.

There exists something cyclical about disease. A single infection goes through several stages in the body from first contact with a host to the pathogen's exit from the body. Outbreaks and epidemics behave in a similar cyclic pattern. A pathogen appears in a community, it takes hold in a few susceptible individuals, and then it spreads by way of various transmission routes.

At their height, outbreaks and epidemics can weaken an entire population of people and make them more susceptible to secondary and opportunistic infections.

The source of a pathogen—this could be a lake, a herd of deer, a cave full of bats, etc.—also influences how disease emerges in your community. Does the pathogen come from a single source such as the Broad Street pump discovered by John Snow? Or does the pathogen come from a thousand or more sources, such as the plague carried by infested rats in the Middle Ages?

The deeper you investigate how infection moves through society, the more fascinating the subject becomes.

The Features of an Infection Outbreak

An outbreak can usually be distinguished from an epidemic because outbreaks affect fewer people and often occur in a specific, confined location.

Outbreaks always arise suddenly and tend to affect a small portion of a population. Thus, outbreaks are usually associated with an infection that arises in a dormitory, a military base, a school, or a section of a town.

Despite the fine distinction between the terms *outbreak* and *epidemic*, or perhaps because of it, epidemiologists increasingly use these terms interchangeably. Even more confusing, some publications have used the term *epidemic outbreak* to, I suppose, cover all their bases.

The CDC shies away from the word *epidemic* and tends to call these events outbreaks, even if they involve hundreds of people. The CDC's decision may be more psychological than scientific. News of an outbreak may be viewed by the public as less serious than an epidemic. In reality, an outbreak of a virulent pathogen poses a bigger heath threat than an epidemic of a less virulent pathogen.

If you like to split hairs, think of an outbreak as a localized epidemic. Remember also that every epidemic begins with either a single local outbreak or a number of local outbreaks in separate places.

Infection Vocabulary

A syndrome is a group of signs, symptoms, lab test results, and changes in a person's behavior or physiology that add up to a specific disease. In other words, a syndrome seems like a combination of diseases that make up one disease.

Examples of infectious syndromes are acquired immunodeficiency syndrome (AIDS) and sudden acute respiratory syndrome (SARS).

Know Your Disease Reservoirs

From where does an outbreak come? Every pathogen has a source. This is the place where the world stores a pathogen until something causes it to enter a human, animal, or plant population. Food, water, soil, people, and the animal kingdom are the main sources of human infection.

A reservoir is also a source of infection. Reservoirs are soil, water, animals, insects, plants, or people in which an infectious agent lives and multiplies when it is not causing infection in a host. Reservoirs are vital to a pathogen's survival because some part of the pathogen's life cycle depends on its reservoir.

You may notice that an infection source and its reservoir seem to be the same thing. In many instances, these two things are indeed the same. Consider a situation that shows how source and reservoir differ. *Cryptosporidium* is a protozoa-like microbe that lives in the digestive tract of many different animal species, such as cattle. Shed with manure, *Cryptosporidium* eventually travels with irrigation water or rainwater into streams and lakes. People usually get a *Cryptosporidium* infection by drinking untreated water. In this example, water is the source of *Cryptosporidium* and cattle serves as its reservoir.

Epidemiologists try to identify the source or reservoir of infection because by blocking people's exposure to it, transmission is also curtailed.

The following list offers examples of known reservoirs of infection:

> ➤ Influenza virus: Swine, waterfowl, and poultry
>
> ➤ Rabies virus: Bats, skunks, foxes, raccoons
>
> ➤ Bubonic plague: Rodents
>
> ➤ Malaria: Monkeys
>
> ➤ Hantavirus: Rodents, mainly deer mice
>
> ➤ Rocky Mountain spotted fever (rickettsia bacteria): Rabbits, squirrels, rats, mice, and groundhogs

Infections and Disease

A zoonotic disease, or zoonosis, is a disease that is communicable between animals and humans. The animals that carry zoonotic disease include wildlife, pets, domesticated farm animals, and exotic animals (zoo animals and imported species such as tropical birds and reptiles).

About 250 microbes are known to cause zoonotic disease. The best example of one is the flu, a disease that starts in swine or birds before moving to humans. When a pathogen goes from one species to another, the action is called a species jump. We tend to forget that species jumps can go in either direction. That is, humans carry germs that on occasion make animals sick.

From Outbreak to Epidemic

An outbreak turns into an epidemic when it spreads to a larger population in a greater area of land. Epidemics therefore affect towns and cities, states, and other geographical regions. In many cases, outbreaks are controllable and epidemics are out of control or much more difficult to control.

A person in authority decides when an outbreak becomes an epidemic. In 2000, a flu outbreak in Britain was discussed in the House of Lords to decide if it should be called an epidemic. The House undoubtedly considered the ramifications of an epidemic on tourism!

Health agencies in Britain, the United States, and elsewhere have put slightly more meaningful constraints on the definition of *epidemic*. Thanks to the reasoning of scientists rather than the posturing of politicians, some diseases have standards to meet to be called an epidemic. An epidemic for disease A might be required to exceed 500 cases per 100,000 people in the population in one week. Disease B might require only 100 cases per 100,000 in a year. Epidemics, therefore, vary by the pathogen that starts them.

So how does an outbreak become a true epidemic? The main way for this to happen is for the outbreak to escape its boundaries. People travel, they go home from college, fly to play a new team, or go on a business trip. This type of movement is the most effective way to turn an outbreak into an epidemic.

Types of Epidemics

Epidemiologists classify epidemics by how they move through a population. The two types of epidemics defined this way are common-source and propagated.

A common-source epidemic enters a population from a single source and reaches a peak in cases in only one to two weeks. Food-borne illnesses are an example of a common-source epidemic.

A propagated epidemic comes from an infected individual who joins a population and initiates a slow, prolonged rise in cases as the infection spreads outward from that person. Propagated epidemics also have more gradual declines than common-source epidemics.

People who are not epidemiologists think of epidemics based on the pathogen that starts the initial infection. For this reason, you are more likely to understand what a flu epidemic is than a propagated epidemic.

Flu Epidemics

Influenza is a unique pathogen. It starts a new epidemic almost every year with a new strain of the influenza virus. Since each year's flu strain can differ quite a bit from those of previous years, influenza also qualifies as an emerging disease as well as a reemerging disease.

The medical community has only limited effectiveness against each year's new flu. Despite impressive efforts to prevent it and the cooperation of health agencies from several nations, the flu always returns and takes its toll.

Flu epidemics usually strike during the winter. The reasons for this seasonality are not completely known. One reason is probably human behavior; people stay indoors in crowded buildings more in winter, and this helps spread the flu germ. You should be aware that flu cases arise sporadically throughout the calendar year and claim several thousand lives in the United States. Furthermore, some strains seem to ignore the winter season completely. For example, the H1N1 flu epidemic of 2009-2010 behaved atypically: it was as common in the summer months as in winter.

The CDC refers to influenza outbreaks as seasonal flu because we think of this disease mainly as a hazard of the cold months. In the northern hemisphere, flu cases begin rising in November to a peak in February, and then decrease in incidence through May.

Flu epidemics move through populations easily, mainly because the virus can spread even if an infected person stands 6 feet away from a susceptible host. Another factor that helps its spread is the fact that an infected person can infect others during the incubation period, before symptoms appear. By the time a carrier realizes that precautions should be taken against transmitting the flu bug, friends and family have probably already caught it. To make matters worse, transmission continues up to one week after the symptoms appear.

Microbe Basics

The flu baffles doctors each year because every year's strains differ a little from those of previous years. Mutagens cause small changes to happen in the substances on the outside of the influenza virus. This makes the virus more difficult to recognize by the immune system.

Antigenic shift is a bigger change inside the virus. In antigenic shift, a virus undergoes a change in its genetic makeup. This leads to a change in the pathogen's behavior, infectivity, or virulence.

In addition to influenza, the AIDS virus also undergoes antigenic drifts and shifts.

Vaccinations may prevent the size of seasonal flu epidemics, but much controversy revolves around the effectiveness of the vaccine. Part of the problem associated with each year's flu vaccine is that it comes from guesswork. Epidemiologists monitor the predominant strains of influenza that seem to be emerging in the coming year. They then select about three of the most likely strains to be health problems the following winter. Scientists devote several months to producing the vaccine, so if the experts have guessed wrong, not enough time will be left to prepare a new, more-effective vaccine.

About 70 million people in the United States are vaccinated against the flu each year. The massive number of flu shots that are administered helps reduce the damage done by this yearly epidemic.

A flu shot alone may not be enough to prevent certain flu strains. Good flu fighting also includes proper hand washing with warm, soapy water for at least twenty seconds while covering all parts of the hands, avoiding touching your face with your hands, and avoiding sick people and crowded places.

The AIDS Epidemic

The medical community learned many things about how infection spreads when the AIDS epidemic arrived. In addition to giving researchers a first-hand case study on propagated epidemics, the AIDS epidemic also gave rise to outbreaks of secondary and opportunistic infections.

The greatest falsehood about AIDS is that the epidemic is over. The AIDS epidemic continues, but it has moved into different age groups, lifestyles, and socioeconomic groups since its emergence in gay men and intravenous drug users in the United States in 1980. (Doctors did not recognize the disease until 1981.)

AIDS is an STD that can also be transmitted by nonsexual methods. Intravenous drug use using contaminated needles, blood transfusions, and hospital accidents have contributed to a portion of the AIDS epidemic.

The AIDS epidemic has been particularly ravaging due to several characteristics of the disease that has hampered its control:

> ➤ The epidemic was slow to be acknowledged by politicians due to the taboos of discussing gay lifestyles, STDs, and drug abuse.

> ➤ Early AIDS patients lost the support of friends, family, and coworkers, leading many to hide their illness.

> ➤ The pathogen destroys the immune system, a bodily system intended to stop infection.

> ➤ Drug treatments developed to slow the infection have been limited in effectiveness and difficult to follow (too many pills given in a complicated daily schedule).

➤ Recently, effective drug treatments have alleviated many symptoms, leading the younger generation to believe AIDS has been cured. (No cure for AIDS currently exists.)

➤ The epidemic has moved into heterosexual populations, requiring a new approach to AIDS education and prevention programs.

Infections in History

The worst epidemics in history took place before epidemiologists existed and used sophisticated surveillance techniques. These epidemics predated antibiotics, vaccines, antiseptics, and good hygiene.

Before microbiology and modern medicine evolved, the worst epidemics belonged to several reoccurrences of bubonic plague. Other serious epidemics since the beginning of recorded history were from syphilis, typhus, smallpox, cholera, yellow fever, and influenza.

Modern epidemics have been caused by dengue fever, mumps, AIDS, measles, and meningitis.

The AIDS epidemic continues to evolve. African-American women represent one of the fastest growing groups to get an HIV infection. In the United States, African-Americans of both sexes account for about half of all HIV infections. A glimmer of good news comes from the fact that new cases have held steady or decreased slightly since the 1990s.

Worldwide, AIDS has grown into a grave problem in regions of middle and low income. In sub-Saharan Africa, one in five adults is infected with HIV. HIV infections are spreading rapidly in parts of Eastern Europe and Central Asia, where the number of people living with AIDS increased more than 50 percent in the last ten years.

When Does HIV Infection Become AIDS?

You may have noticed I talk about HIV infection and the disease AIDS almost interchangeably. The initial infection with HIV begins a slow progression toward disease. This is characteristic of a latent disease, one that can take years before symptoms develop. Because no cure exists for AIDS, an HIV infection has long been tantamount to developing a full-blown case of AIDS.

Today, a diagnosis of the disease includes the following guidelines:

➤ HIV infection with a CD4+ T-cell count of less than 200 per milliliter

➤ HIV infection with CD4+ T-cells accounting for less than 14 percent of all lymphocytes

➤ HIV infection with at least one of twenty-two secondary or opportunistic infections

Because of the slow progression of HIV infection to AIDS, medical professionals now tend to refer to this disease as HIV/AIDS. The symptoms of the disease AIDS include the above hallmarks plus neurological disorders (dementia, anxiety), possible insomnia, depression, and wasting disease. Wasting disease is a progressive loss of muscle and fat tissue.

Infections in History

In total numbers of victims and also in the percent of the population affected, the Black Death ranks as the worst epidemic in humanity's history. The Black Death was one of several recurrences of bubonic plague, a bacterial disease so called because of the blood vessel hemorrhages it causes underneath the skin, leaving dark bruise-like patches.

The Black Death arrived in Europe in 1347 by way of trade routes through Central Asia from the Far East. Rodents carrying the pathogen *Yersinia pestis* would have been bitten by fleas, which in turn transmitted the plague to people with their bites. The Black Death consumed all of Europe from the Atlantic to the Ural Mountains for the next three years when it died out on its own.

By its end, the epidemic had killed between a quarter and a third of Europe's population. It devastated every segment of society and so had lasting effects on the arts, medicine, education, politics, and financial systems. The Black Death contributed to the death of the feudal system of land ownership and changed forever how the clergy would lead their communities.

Few people today realize that bubonic plague persists. Despite sporadic outbreaks, the overwhelming plagues that haunted the Middle Ages never returned with the same ferocity. Improved hygiene, community sanitation, pest control, and antibiotics may have consigned the bubonic plague to the back pages of our stories on epidemics.

Other Modern Epidemics

AIDS and the yearly flu outbreaks may be the best-known epidemics that we confront today. In certain regions of the world, however, other infections reach epidemic proportions. Many pathogens cause recurring epidemics in places where poverty has reduced medicine's ability to reach people to diagnose disease, give drugs, and provide other treatments.

The World Health Organization (WHO) has identified the following infectious diseases as currently in epidemic proportions or expected to recur in the near future:

➤ Bubonic plague: The plague recurs in epidemic form almost yearly in Africa, Asia, and South America. Some of these events are small. Peru's epidemic outbreak of 2010 affected seventeen people. They were thought to have caught the pathogen from domestic cats, rodents, or other people.

➤ Dengue fever: This infection is caused by a mosquito-borne virus. Like many mosquito-borne infections, dengue fever cases increase in the tropics or subtropical areas. The disease causes mild to severe fever, rash, headaches, and various pains. Dengue can be fatal; no treatments are available for it. Epidemics occur yearly in Central Asia.

➤ Cholera: Cholera is an intestinal infection and severe diarrheal disease caused by ingesting water or food contaminated with *Vibrio cholerae* bacteria. Epidemics are most likely to occur when a natural disaster, such as a typhoon, causes flooding. Water treatment systems and food distribution tend to be overwhelmed in these conditions and contaminated. Cholera causes several thousand deaths worldwide annually. Cholera can occur anywhere other than the polar regions but is most prevalent in sub-Saharan Africa, Asia, and Southeast Asia. Using clean water is the best prevention for cholera. Vaccines for cholera are limited, although travelers to cholera-affected parts of the world can ask their doctor for an oral vaccine.

➤ Meningitis: Bacterial, viral, and fungal forms of this disease cause inflammation of the membranes that line the brain and spinal cord (the meninges). Bacterial meningitis appears in sporadic outbreaks worldwide almost every year. An area of sub-Saharan Africa from Senegal to Ethiopia has been called the meningitis belt. In this region, several thousand deaths occur yearly. If untreated, bacterial meningitis kills one out of every two people infected. A vaccine against the main bacterial pathogen *Neisseria meningitidis* was introduced in 2010, but most countries in need have not yet received a supply of this new drug.

➤ Typhoid (typhoid fever): This bacterial infection caused by *Salmonella typhi* is transmitted through food and water contaminated with fecal matter. Infected people suffer the common symptoms of food-borne illness—fever, headache, nausea, diarrhea, and weakness. The most serious recent outbreaks have occurred in the Democratic Republic of the Congo and Haiti. A 2004 epidemic in Africa reached almost 45,000 cases and caused more than 200 deaths. Antibiotic treatment is the main approach to halting a typhoid epidemic.

➤ STDs, also called sexually transmitted infections (STIs): More than thirty different pathogens cause STDs. In some developing countries, at least one STD outbreak occurs almost every year. Over 300 million cases are reported worldwide. The most common STDs to reach epidemic proportions are syphilis, gonorrhea, chlamydia, and trichomoniasis.

Infections in History

The patterns of infectious disease change as society changes. As long as a disease does not wipe out a population as the Black Death and AIDS have threatened to do six centuries apart, humans learn to coexist with their pathogens.

Some changes in society can, however, change the patterns of disease outbreak and expand the spread of infection. The main factors that catch the eye of epidemiologists are the following:

➤ The emergence of new pathogens to populations that have no resistance to it, which is caused in part by immigration.

➤ Increased urbanization, the shift in where people live from rural homes to cities, increases population density and helps diseases like TB spread.

➤ Unending wars, famine, and poverty put people at heightened risk for infection. This comes about due to malnutrition, injuries, and increased susceptibility.

➤ Increases in risky sexual behavior have kept STDs at or near epidemic proportions.

➤ Factory farming, the large-scale production of meat, dairy products, eggs, and fish, help pathogens concentrate. Global distribution of these foods plus fresh produce also spread food germs far and wide.

➤ Development of previously undisturbed land puts people closer to pathogen reservoirs, such as rodents, birds, and other wildlife.

➤ The unabated increase in antibiotic resistance among pathogens helps keep infections in our population.

CHAPTER 10

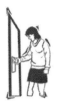

Contact and Vehicle Transmission

In This Chapter

➤ Defining the three types of contact transmission

➤ Explaining how indirect contact transmission works

➤ Comparing indirect germ transmission and vehicle transmission

➤ Learning the ways to "see" germs on objects around us

This chapter will remind you of the importance of knowing how germs are transmitted so that you can make sound decisions on how to block transmission. It focuses on the two most common ways people in the United States get infections. One is through contact with another living thing that is carrying germs. The other method involves touching a nonliving object that also carries germs.

It seems there is nowhere to turn where germs won't find you! That may be true, but to fight infection you might consider changing your way of thinking about germs. Rather than let germs come to you, be constantly aware of these invisible invaders. Note every object around you that might carry germs and you pick them up voluntary. Have I just described a germophobe? Perhaps so, but if you're serious about decreasing the number of infections you and your loved ones get each year, a little germophobia doesn't hurt.

Contact Transmission

Contact transmission is person-to-person transmission. This type of transmission is the most effective way to share germs: simply deposit a load of microbes directly onto the body of another person. If a friend, lover, or stranger puts their germs on you, I hope your resistance is up to snuff. Otherwise, your chance of infection increases with each stumble in your first-, second-, and third-line defenses.

For contact transmission to successfully transfer germs from one person to the next, you do not always have to touch another person. Touching works best, but a very close association with another person transmits germs almost as effectively. That's why epidemiologists divide contact transmission into three types:

➤ Directly touching another person

➤ Sharing an inanimate object

➤ Exchanging germs through the air

Infections in History

Throughout most of human history, infectious disease was thought to be caused by supernatural forces on Earth or in the heavens. Society attributed infections to miasma, a poisonous vapor that infiltrates the body. The clergy were quick to point out that miasma was more apt to strike sinners than those close to God.

The rejection of the miasma theory and the acceptance of microbes as the cause of infection represent a monumental achievement in science. Dozens of biologists contributed to our knowledge of the microbe-infection connection, and their work spanned centuries.

The first person to realize that microscopic germs were responsible for infection was Hungarian physician Ignaz Semmelweis. In the mid-1800s, he began the then-unheard-of practice of washing his hands before delivering babies. Infections in women giving birth soon decreased. Sadly, his colleagues dismissed his germ theory and he suffered depression late in his career. In cruel irony, Semmelweis died from an infected wound.

Direct Contact Transmission

Direct contact transmission of pathogens occurs when people touch and an infected individual passes germs to a healthy individual. The most common actions in transmission are touching, kissing, and sexual intercourse. The last two put pathogens on mucous membranes rather than on skin, and you've already learned that these membranes lack the stout resistance against infection that skin possesses. The chances of infection increase in any type of transmission if you have an injury to the skin that weakens its ability to keep microbes out of your body.

Infections and Disease

Infectious mononucleosis is an acute infection caused by the Epstein-Barr virus. Most prevalent in the age group of fifteen to twenty-five years, this infection causes abnormally high levels of white blood cells called mononuclear leukocytes. After age twenty-five, people develop resistance to infection.

Known colloquially as the kissing disease, infectious mononucleosis is transmitted in saliva. The virus first infects the cells lining the pharynx and salivary glands then spreads to lymph nodes, the spleen, and the liver by hiding inside the body's circulating lymphocytes. This disease's incubation period lasts thirty to forty-five days, illness lasts up to four weeks, and the disease usually goes away on its own.

Direct contact also includes sharing body secretions, even if for some reason no touching takes place, and touching an infected animal, including pets. Several dermatophytoses (fungal infections of the skin surface) can be caught from dogs, cats, rats, mice, hamsters, guinea pigs, reptiles, and amphibians. A wider variety of more serious infections can occur when the human-animal contact involves a bite, scratch, or contamination by the oral-fecal route of transmission.

Keep in mind that animals transmit two general types of pathogens. One is a pathogen that uses the animal as a reservoir. For example, a bite from a rabid fox will lead to the rabies disease. The other example involves situations where an animal carries a pathogen from place to place; a kind of physical conveyance. Picture your dog coming home from a happy romp at the town dump.

Some of the common infections transmitted by direct person-to-person contact are the STDs, nonsexually transmitted herpes, boils, colds, flu, measles, scarlet fever, infectious mononucleosis, and staph infections. Diseases passed through the placenta from mother to infant (AIDS and syphilis) also fall into this category. Finally, infections passed from a mother to a nursing child can be classified as direct contact transmissions.

Microbe Basics

The oral-fecal route of transmission means ingesting (accidently, I hope) feces filled with pathogens. Yes, it's as disgusting as it sounds and is a very common way to get sick.

People help oral-fecal transmission immensely by touching their germ-carrying fingers to their face, especially the mucous membranes of the eye, nose, and mouth.

Microbiologists using hidden cameras have watched adults and children touch their faces. Adults touch their hands to their face one to three times every five minutes. That adds up to thousands of touches in a waking day. Children do it three times more frequently.

To fight infection, assume everyone else is not as conscientious about personal hygiene as you are. Every person represents a potential mother lode of germs, most of them straight from the bathroom. Are you less inclined to touch your face now? I thought so.

Indirect Contact Transmission

Indirect contact transmission involves an inanimate object that bridges the gap between an infected person and a healthy person. In these cases, the people are close but not touching.

Shared bedding, towels, eating utensils, drinking cups, water bottles, lip balm, thermometers, and toothbrushes provide examples of shared items of an intimate nature that help move germs around. Drug abusers who share needles transmit pathogens this way.

Indirect contact transmission resembles vehicle transmission, to be discussed shortly. In both types of transmission, the inanimate object that carries a pathogen from one person to another is called a fomite.

Droplet Transmission

Droplet transmission spreads germs via sneezing, coughing, laughing, animated talking, and spitting, all of which produce small droplets of saliva. These droplets contain a varying amount of mucus and microbes.

Most droplets travel no more than a few feet, but a person can produce a large number in a short period of time. One sneeze can expel 20,000 droplets!

Picture a holiday office party in December. Flu season is peaking. You've been working overtime for weeks to make a year-end deadline, so you're run down, stressed, and have been subsisting on pigs in a blanket from the hors d'oeurves tray. A cough here, a sneeze there, and the guy in your face insists on telling a bawdy joke at top volume. Is there any doubt droplet transmission will spread the virus throughout this gathering? No.

Microbe Basics

Porous materials such as wood, cement, granite, caulking, and fabric provide more hiding places for microbes than hard surfaces (glass, tile, porcelain, and metal). For this reason, people have viewed wooden cutting boards as a place that entraps infection-causing microbes from raw meats, fish, and fresh produce.

Plastic cutting boards became popular several years ago as a safer alternative to wood. Many plastic cutting boards have an antimicrobial chemical (usually triclosan) as an added boost for repelling microbes.

Microbiologists have launched dozens of studies on the wood versus plastic question. They found that both types of cutting boards hold plenty of microbes in the fissures made by knives. Plastic cutting boards were actually harder to clean in soap and water than the wooden kind. Chemically treated plastic cutting boards furthermore give only a false sense of security. A raw chicken releases enough *Salmonella* on a cutting board, treated or not, to make a family sick.

The key to cutting board care is to follow three rules:

➤ Use separate boards, one for raw meats, another for fresh vegetables and fruits

➤ Wash all cutting boards thoroughly after each use by scrubbing with warm, soapy water

➤ Following liberal rinsing in clean water, let the boards dry completely before using them again

Infections in addition to colds and flu that transmit via droplets are whooping cough, pneumonia, measles, and—rabies! The rabies virus has been known to occur when a person enters an area dense with roosting bats, such as a cave. The virus is in the bats' saliva and can be inhaled using droplet transmission. This is rare but it happens.

Vehicle Transmission

Vehicle transmission resembles indirect contact transmission in that they both use an inanimate object to pass germs among people. I distinguish these two forms of transmission as follows:

> ➤ Indirect contact transmission involves intimately shared items with little time between germ deposit and germ pickup.

> ➤ Vehicle transmission involves common objects repeatedly touched by many people, usually strangers, with longer time periods between germ deposit and germ pickup.

Microbe Basics

Scientific studies on the number of bacteria and fungi in households consistently find the highest numbers in the following places, roughly in order from highest to lowest:

➤ Kitchen drain

➤ Shower drain

➤ Kitchen sponge

➤ Kitchen garbage can

➤ Refrigerator handle

➤ Toilet bowl

➤ Bathroom doorknob

➤ Cutting board

Assorted other handles and buttons on the microwave, dishwasher, garbage can cabinet or lid, and toilet flush handle can harbor a lot of germs as can countertops, the kitchen table, pet areas, and children's playrooms and toys.

The stuff growing on what used to be a piece of fruit in your refrigerator may look gruesome, but it poses less of a threat than foods you'll actually eat. Foods represent a separate category of germ carrier and are usually not included in discussions on vehicle transmission.

Vehicle transmission can certainly happen among friends and family—we'll visit the kitchen in a moment to see how—but it also involves transmission among the public. Somehow, getting pathogens from strangers scares germophobes more than pathogens from loved ones, but you get sick either way.

Microbes are everywhere and a certain small percent of them on any surface could be pathogenic. During cold and flu season the percentage of pathogens probably goes up. Though any surface can carry pathogens, two hallmarks of vehicle transmission always seem to hold true: more pathogens are found on items touched by people's hands than any other part of their body, and moisture on the item helps transmission.

The first point regarding hands is true even for bathrooms. More than one microbiologist has pointed out that bathrooms are safer than kitchens in regard to transmission. I'll give you an image to ponder. You have a better chance of getting sick by licking a refrigerator handle than by licking a toilet seat. (But I don't recommend doing either.)

Common Vehicles in the Home

Microbiologists study households for their so-called germ hot spots. Regardless of your devotion to housecleaning or the type of foods you cook, the same hot spots emerge in almost every home. These are the kitchen and the bathroom, usually in that order. Other parts of the house vary depending on whether someone at home is sick and whether you have children or pets.

Most of the studies on germ hot spots focus on bacteria, but viruses and fungi occupy your home too. Viruses follow much the same pattern of distribution as bacteria, that is they hang around in kitchens and bathrooms. Molds tend to congregate in dusty places, such as closets, in curtains, and on upholstered furniture. Mildew is common in bathrooms.

Common sense should tell you where most germs lurk in the home. They are found on any surface repeatedly touched by several people. They are also prevalent on surfaces that touch food. The grocery bag is in fact one of the most germ-dense things you bring into your house other than the soles of your shoes.

Common Vehicles in Work and on the Way to Work

Famous microbiologist Charles Gerba once said, "The only time people clean their desk at work is when they start sticking to it." An argument can be made that the workplace outdistances all other sites for transmitting germs. Think about the factors that come together to make a perfect storm for workplace germs:

➤ Several shared surfaces never get cleaned

➤ People come into work sick

➤ Uninfected workers are stressed by inadequate sleep and poor nutrition choices (Do you choose a doughnut or the fresh fruit at staff meetings?)

➤ Enclosed buildings with suboptimal ventilation

➤ Carpool vans or public transportation expose you to germs before you even make it to work

Workplace hot spots for germs tend to be computer keyboards, especially shared computers, the computer mouse, vending machine buttons, and, in fact, all buttons—microwave, copier, fax machine, elevator, phone, etc.

The hotel rooms you stay at on business trips may look clean, but they are gnarly hot spots. The TV remote, the game console control, bedspreads, the desk, and faucet handles carry a variety of microbes. Rooms that look clean may have as many if not more germs than dirty-looking rooms. This is due to the cleaning rags used by the hotel housekeepers. They rarely get adequate cleaning and the disinfectants may have been diluted beyond their usefulness by the time a person gets around to your room. On a happy note, phones used to be thought of as a germ vehicle, but the use of personal cell phones may have turned the hotel room phone into one of its cleanest items.

Any conveyance that uses the word *public* can be assumed to hold germs. Public transportation is rife with shared surfaces touched hundreds of times by hundreds of people between cleanings. On airplanes shared surfaces include tray tables, pillows, blankets, seats, armrests, in-flight magazines, and virtually every surface in the restroom. On other forms of public transportation, beware of poles, railings, overhead straps, and door handles.

Infections and Disease

Almost everyone would name public restrooms as a potential hot spot of pathogens. These places get a workout; lots of shared surfaces and lots of fecal microbes. Other than avoiding these places altogether, you cannot make public restrooms into germ-safe environments. But you can reduce the chance of infection by doing the following:

➤ Choose the first stall on the right, which tends to get less action

➤ In dirty restrooms, choose the cleanest-looking stall possible and make sure the seat appears clean

➤ Minimize the number of surfaces you touch with your hands while inside the stall

➤ Do not put your handbag, briefcase, or backpack on the floor

➤ Leave the stall as quickly as possible after flushing to avoid airborne moisture droplets

➤ Wash your hands thoroughly before leaving the restroom

➤ Use a paper towel to open the door when leaving.

Common Vehicles in Schools

Schools today are like offices with crayons. The nooks and crannies of school computer keyboards carry as many microbes as the keyboard downtown. The same surfaces occur in school cafeterias as in office cafeterias. The same goes for the gym and locker room.

The age of your child will give you an idea of the most probable forms of germ sharing. In day care, toddlers spend lots of time on the floor, put toys and other objects into their mouths, and wear diapers. Vehicle transmission is rampant. Indeed, outbreaks of rotavirus diarrhea and other ailments that transmit via the oral-fecal route are common in day care centers.

Older children have a better idea about hygiene and hand washing. They might nevertheless forget about the germ hot spots in their exuberance to get to recess. Hot spots include water fountains, vending machines, library materials, and desks.

In the teenager's world, things change again. The same shared surfaces exist, but now a parent has to wonder about the other goings-on, such as hand holding, hugging, kissing, and sharing water bottles, cosmetics, and clothes.

In college, we have the unnatural situation of a hundred strangers getting little sleep and terrible food, packed into a building they call the dorm. Cold, flu, and other outbreaks are especially common on college campuses. Transmission occurs by direct and indirect contact, droplets, and vehicles, probably in about equal amounts.

Germ Transmission in Hospitals

Hospitals are danger zones for germ transmission because of the high concentration of both pathogens and a susceptible population of patients. Do not overlook the possible transmission routes in hospitals.

Hospitals have a high occurrence of direct, indirect, and droplet transmission plus potential germs on a diversity of medical instruments. For nurses, doctors, and aides to do their job, they must get close to patients, touch them, and use medical instruments. Many of these instruments are invasive, meaning they go into the patient's body cavities or under the skin.

Health care workers often make extraordinary efforts to give their patients the best care possible. Yet recent studies showed an alarming lack of good hygiene among these professionals. Less than half the doctors and nurses wash their hands between patients. Many do not wash their hands properly. The word has gone out to the health care industry about this problem and, hopefully, hygiene habits have improved. Even in the best of circumstances, however, hospitals are places with an increased chance of germ transmission.

Infection Vocabulary

Sharps is the nickname health care workers give to items that cause cuts or punctures in the skin. Sharps include syringes with needles, scalpels, blades and razors, suture needles, and broken glassware. These items present an increased risk of transmitting pathogens because they are intended to break the skin barrier and come in contact with underlying connective tissue or blood.

Sharps create two types of transmission hazards: patient-to-patient transfer with contaminated sharps and patient-to-health care worker transmission of a pathogen. The second more common hazard involving sharps relates to medical waste. Sharps sometimes get into the environment by escaping from landfills. If the item is contaminated with an infectious agent, it can be a means of transmitting infection to people, pets, or wildlife.

The Germs Around Us

You know the feeling. You accidentally drop a cookie on the floor. Should you pick it up and pop it in your mouth as if nothing happened? Or should you assume your favorite homemade chocolate chip cookie is now a festering ball of mayhem?

Your comfort level in coexisting with the germs around you relates to your degree of germophobia. A germophobe would never ingest any piece of food that had touched the floor or a restaurant table, kitchen counter, or desk at the office. More likely, you assess the situation. Does the floor look clean or is it a filthy thoroughfare? Give yourself credit for the common sense you call upon each time something like this happens.

Kids and plenty of adults call on the five-second rule to help them navigate the world of germs. The rule says that if you picked up a piece of food within five seconds after dropping it, it's still safe to eat because germs haven't had time to attach to the morsel. Rather than pull out a stopwatch, reach for your common sense. Surfaces in your clean home pose less of a threat of transmitting germs than the floor at Grand Central Station. But even at home, a crumb that has landed on your kitchen floor carries less possibility for infection if picked up right away than a crumb that has been there since last month!

Remember also that moist surfaces are always more likely to contain infectious germs than dry surfaces. A messy, wet kitchen counter doesn't sound safer to me than a corner of your living room that gets little traffic.

Psychology plays a part, too. Scientists have discovered that people apply the five-second rule differently to different foods. If a piece of brownie is dropped, most people throw caution to the wind and pick it up and enjoy. Did a piece of broccoli earn the same reverence? Not so much.

CHAPTER 11

Airborne and Vector Transmission

In This Chapter

➤ Describing airborne transmission and comparing to droplet transmission

➤ Describing the way bioaerosols move through air

➤ Listing important airborne pathogens of humans

➤ Describing types of vehicles in vehicle transmission

➤ Examining the way vectors transmit infection

➤ Describing the major vector-control programs

In this chapter we complete our examination of the various modes of infection transmission. The topics are airborne transmission and vector transmission.

Airborne Transmission

Pathogens use airborne transmission to infect hosts far away from the pathogen's source. The advantages to a pathogen are obvious. Airborne transmission allows an infectious agent to spread further through a population than would be possible if limited to person-to-person contact. Conversely, airborne transmission makes things more difficult for you in preventing infection because you have no way of knowing if a pathogen is coming your way.

Airborne transmission differs from the droplet type of contact transmission by the distance airborne pathogens travel. In airborne transmission, a pathogen travels several feet to more than a mile compared to a few feet for droplet transmission.

Specific bacteria, viruses, and fungi use airborne travel for finding a host to infect. In addition, several microbial toxins move through the air. Yet these microbes do not multiply in the air. The air is a mode of transportation, but the pathogen still must infect a living thing to make new generations.

Plant diseases rely almost exclusively on airborne transmission and transport by insects or animals. Plant pathogens would by necessity have evolved to use airborne travel since plants and trees can't move around like other hosts can. Some rust infections, for example, travel from Texas to the Dakotas on prevailing winds.

Aeromicrobiology is the study of microbes in the atmosphere. Microbiologists in this specialty focus on tiny airborne moisture packets called bioaerosols. The *bio* part of the word means these packets contain something biological, usually a microbe or a toxin.

Very few microbes travel through air alone. Most go airborne inside miniscule particles such as bioaerosols, saliva droplets, dust, or dirt. Two exceptions are pollen and fungal spores, which are designed to stay aloft and travel long distances in the atmosphere.

Infection Vocabulary

Aeromicrobiology is a new area of study in microbiology, and it's concerned with the types and numbers of microbes in air. This subject includes the number of pathogens in the air, how they get there, the distance they travel between reservoir and host, and the physics involved in propelling microbes into the air and then settling to earth.

Bioaerosols and How the Wind Blows

An entire science is devoted to how bioaerosols take off from their launch site, drift on the breeze, and settle out of air by gravity. For infection fighting, the physics of bioaerosol movement isn't as important to know as the following basics of airborne transport:

> Bioaerosols carry infection only if they can keep the microbe inside them alive or the toxin infectious. Air is normally an inhospitable place for microbes because it dries out the cells, and microbes are vulnerable to damage by radiation and oxygen chemicals in the higher atmosphere, such as ozone.

> Pathogens survive in the air longer at higher relative humidity and die faster at lower relative humidity. No microbe can survive for long without moisture.

> High temperatures and freezing temperatures both decrease the survivability of pathogens in the air.

> Certain occupations produce a large number of pathogen-containing bioaerosols. Construction sites, hospitals, and microbiology labs have been blamed for putting bioaerosols into the atmosphere.

Bioaerosols move through the air and settle out of air more like a feather than a cannonball. Wind speed and air turbulence determine how bioaerosols reach you. In almost all instances of infection, bioaerosols use the respiratory tract as their portal of entry. Therefore, the main diseases that involve airborne transmission begin as an infection in which the pathogen had been inhaled.

Important Airborne Infections

Humans, animals, and plants are all susceptible to airborne pathogens. The main airborne infections in people are the following:

> TB: Caused by *Mycobacterium tuberculosis*

> Influenza: Caused by the flu virus

> Pneumonia: Caused by the bacteria *Klebsiella pneumoniae* and *Legionella pneumophila*, and the fungus *Pneumocystis jiroveci*

> Whooping cough: Caused by the bacterium *Bordetella pertussis*

> The common cold: Caused by rhinovirus and coronavirus

> Diphtheria: Caused by the bacterium *Corynebacterium diphtheriae*

Infections in History

A new disease emerged in Philadelphia in the summer of 1976 during a Legionnaires' convention. Victims suffered with headaches and fever, which progressed to life-threatening pneumonia.

The new pathogen would be named *Legionella pneumophila. L. pneumophila* is a microbe that lives in water, but infection is transmitted when the cells become aerosolized in moisture droplets and the bioaerosols are inhaled. In the 1976 outbreak, the fateful bioaerosols had been dispersed by the convention hotel's air conditioning and ventilation system.

Microbiologists now recognize *L. pneumophila* as one of several major causes of pneumonia.

Vector-Borne Transmission

Vector-borne transmission is the spread of infection by way of an arthropod (mites, ticks, flies, fleas, and other insects) or a vertebrate (dogs, cats, bats, wildlife, and livestock). Vertebrate transmission also qualifies as a zoonotic disease, so in this chapter I'll cover only vectors that are insects. Insects are the largest and most diverse group of transmission vectors known.

The WHO recognizes vector-borne transmission as a major route of disease transmission worldwide. For this reason, many countries have vector-control programs for blocking transmission to susceptible populations. Unfortunately, vector control has proven to be extremely difficult. Some of the factors that are thought to affect vector breeding and populations are as follows:

➤ Climate change leads to abnormally violent storms and flooding, affecting the breeding seasons and populations of insects.

➤ Deforestation has increased flooding and standing water, which are breeding grounds for mosquitoes.

➤ Global warming might change the reproductive cycles of many insects.

➤ Biodiversity loss impacts the species that normally prey on insects.

The factors listed here show that vector control is a global issue, not easily solved. Insects migrate. Global shipping and air travel also expand the range of insect vectors. Thus, vector control will be an ongoing issue in infection control for some time to come.

Types of Vector-Borne Transmission

Insects can carry pathogens either inside their bodies or stuck on their bodies. Microbiologists who devote careers extracting pathogens from insects have therefore developed different categories based on how vectors carry pathogens. These also give epidemiologists three subcategories of vector transmission:

➤ Mechanical transmission: The pathogen sticks to the outside of the insect and passively rides along to wherever the insect goes. An example of mechanical transmission is when flies carry *E. coli* from garbage to a picnic table.

➤ Biological transmission: The pathogen goes through at least one stage in its life cycle inside the insect and needs the insect to survive. The malaria pathogen uses biological transmission.

➤ Harborage transmission: The pathogen spends time inside the insect but doesn't undergo any life cycle changes. The plague pathogen, *Yersinia pestis*, spends time inside fleas before moving on to rats or a human host.

Arthropods and Infection

Arthropod-borne infections tend to be more prevalent in the tropics than in the world's temperate regions. Most of these infections come from biting insects.

Biting insects (flies, ticks, fleas, etc.) transmit pathogens in their saliva to the host organism's blood or, more rarely, mucous membranes. People may think of biting insects as blood-sucking pests, but the first step in the transmission process is an injection of saliva into the host rather than a withdrawal of the host's blood. The saliva of several insect species contains an anticoagulant that prevents the blood from clotting. By preventing this natural reaction of the host's defenses, the insect enhances its chance to get a meal. It is during the injection of saliva that the pathogen gains entry to the host.

Infections and Disease

In a lifetime, mosquitoes might meander only a few yards from where they hatch. But they often find their way onto airplanes, oceangoing ships, trains, cars, and trucks. As a result, mosquito-borne diseases can spread far from the tropical areas where they are endemic.

Airlines use insecticide sprays to kill mosquitoes and other insect stowaways, which blocks some of the long-distance travel of mosquitoes. But these insects continue to travel on oceangoing ships, on trains, in cars, and on animals and people.

More than 3,000 species of mosquitoes are known to exist. Scientists probably have identified only a fraction that can carry disease. In human health, three genera pose definite health risks. Species of the genus *Anopheles* are the only ones known to carry malaria. *Anopheles* also carries pathogens that cause eliphantiasis and various forms of encephalitis. *Culex* species also carry encephalitis viruses plus the West Nile virus. *Aedes* mosquitoes carry the viruses that cause yellow fever, dengue fever, and additional forms of encephalitis.

National and local public health agencies put considerable efforts into mosquito control by spraying breeding areas in summer. This vector nevertheless remains a significant threat to world health.

The following are the important arthropods that transmit infections to humans by biting:

➤ Mosquitoes: Dengue fever, encephalitis, filariasis, malaria, Rift Valley fever, tularemia, West Nile virus, yellow fever; also pet disease such as heartworm in dogs

➤ Ticks: Anaplasmosis, babesiosis, Colorado tick fever, ehrlichiosis, Lyme disease, Mediterranean fever, relapsing fever (also by lice), Rocky Mountain spotted fever

> ➤ Fleas: Bubonic plague, typhus fever
>
> ➤ Flies: African sleeping sickness (trypanosomiasis transmitted by tsetse fly), leishmaniasis (sandflies), river blindness (black flies)
>
> ➤ Mites: Scrub fever

Although vaccines are available for some of the infections listed above, vector control programs have received more attention for stopping vector-borne transmission. I'll cover the reasons and the main types of programs later in this chapter.

Flies

Flies transmit pathogens either by biting a host or by using mechanical transmission to transport pathogens. Flies may be the insect vector most closely associated with mechanical transmission. In addition, flies are widespread and not reliant on tropical regions for maintaining their populations.

Picture a fly grazing through a dumpster, buzzing inside a Porta Potty, and then heading in the direction of your Fourth of July picnic. Although almost impossible to prove, microbiologists know this mode of transmission occurs often. The prevention for this type of transmission is simple: cover foods with plastic wrap or keep in closed containers, store in the refrigerator until just before serving, and put away in the refrigerator immediately after a meal.

Mechanical transmission by flies probably contributes to a portion of the incidence of cholera, hepatitis A, typhoid, giardiasis, amoebiasis, rotavirus infection, polio, and typhoid. Flies have also been implicated in the transmission of diarrheal diseases (probably from food-borne pathogens), anthrax, eye infections, and TB. The fly-infection link has been difficult to prove through science, but easy to imagine.

Infections and Disease

In the United States, ticks are a major vector in transmitting infection. Tick-borne diseases have several characteristic symptoms in common, including fever, chills, muscle aches, headache, fatigue, and different types of rashes. The appearance and pattern of each rash are, in fact, used by doctors to diagnose tick infections. For example, a spotty rash may indicate Rocky Mountain spotted fever; an ulcer-related rash indicates tularemia.

Since different species of tick live in certain regions of North America, doctors use the geographic location, rash features, and unique symptoms to diagnose tick-borne infections.

Vector Control

A personal vector-control program means you put on insect-repelling clothing or apply a chemical repellent. Staying indoors during the peak time for mosquitoes and putting screens on doors and windows provide straightforward ways to keep biting insects away from you.

International health organizations have rolled out broader vector-control programs. These approaches aim at affecting the breeding populations of mosquitoes and other insects. You may notice one aspect of local vector control when in the summer you see trucks spraying insecticides rumble through wooded neighborhoods. Following are other vector-control steps:

➤ Blanket spraying or fogging of insecticides on breeding grounds such as wetlands and woods

➤ Woodland clearing to reduce breeding grounds

➤ Use of insecticide-treated mosquito nets

➤ Application of biological control programs, such as microbial pathogens that infect the insects

➤ Encouragement of predator species (birds, bats, reptiles, etc.)

➤ Filtering water sources to remove larvae

➤ Trapping

➤ Use of sterilization chemicals

Vector-control programs generate concern among some biologists because insects serve as a food for birds, reptiles, amphibians, and other insects. Biologists must balance the desire to control infectious diseases with the need to sustain Earth's diversity of species.

PART THREE

Preventing Infection Transmission

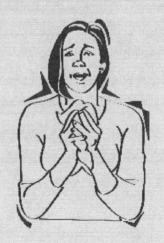

CHAPTER 12

Controlling Disease Transmission Routes

In this chapter you'll receive practical advice on how to control disease transmission routes. Having learned about contact transmission, vectors, and other ways in which pathogens get from their source to a host, we now wish to block those routes to prevent infection.

The most effective way to avoid germ transmission is to stay far away from other people, animals, soil, and suspect foods and water. This is neither practical nor possible.

We take certain actions that we've learned can make it more difficult for pathogens to move from place to place. Most important, these actions keep germs from finding you. They include frequent hand washing, especially before handling food and after using restrooms, avoiding others who show signs of being sick, and keeping the hands away from the face.

Another step in preventing transmission involves good housekeeping. This means keeping your surroundings clean so that germs do not accumulate on surfaces.

Let's look at what *clean* really means. How do we know we've removed germs from surfaces if germs are invisible? You may not want to use harsh cleaners in your home, especially around kids and pets. This chapter helps you make the right decisions for fighting infection without living in a soup of chemical products.

The Meaning of *Clean*

How do you know when pathogens are on your desk, countertop, or floor? Sometimes it's easy. If your spouse is staying home sick with a cold, walks into the kitchen, and sneezes onto your toast, you can be confident the toast now holds a large dose of viruses. In most other times, spotting germs is not as straightforward.

Start hunting germs by assessing your surroundings. I like to say that you may not always see dirt, but you can always see filth. The cleanliness of any home, office, or dorm room tells a story and just might give you a clue to your chances of getting an infection.

Dirt ranges from microscopic particles to large, visible chunks of soil, food, and unidentified yuck. Microscopic bits of dust are as likely to carry thousands of microbes as a large piece of yuck. That's because all dirt gives microbes a place to hide. When a nurse advises you to clean a cut on the skin with soap and clear water, this message is not about the dirt but about the microbes clinging to the dirt.

Dirt works the same way in homes and in offices: it hides germs in a safe location until the microbes can move to a susceptible host. As cozy as this clump may be, a pathogen's ultimate goal is to get inside a host that offers a warm home, nutrients, water, and other factors that promote growth. Cleaning that removes visible dirt is therefore a good start toward reducing the germs in your surroundings.

Microbe Basics

Sterilization is the removal of all living things from a material. This means the elimination of all types of microbes in addition to bacterial spores. Most grocery stores do not sell chemical sterilants. These products are used more frequently by hospitals and other healthcare settings.

Manufacturers wishing to advertise their products on TV make a list of the benefits the product will give to consumers. These benefits are called claims. By familiarizing yourself with the claims on cleaning products, you can make better purchases when looking for a product to kill the flu virus, *E. coli*, or other hazards.

Here is a primer on the three main types of cleaning products you can buy. All of the following products are for use only on inanimate surfaces and are not to be used on the body.

> ➤ Cleaners: Products that remove dirt from inanimate surfaces but probably do not kill germs

> ➤ Disinfectants: Products that kill all germs

> ➤ Sanitizers: Products that reduce the number of germs present on a surface to safe levels

Infection Vocabulary

An antiseptic is a different type of product intended to remove germs from the skin. Some antiseptics, like rubbing alcohol and hydrogen peroxide, can be used in a pinch to clean up a spot of something you think holds germs, but that is not the main job of antiseptics.

Cleaners

Cleaners or cleansers are products that remove large amounts of dirt from inanimate materials. When the dirt disappears, it takes lots of microbes with it. Various cleaners are formulated to remove grease, food, soap scum, and other types of grime, but we cannot be sure of the amount of microbes they eliminate. Unlike disinfectants and sanitizers, cleaners are not tested to determine the types and amounts of microbes they kill.

Reading the Cleaner's Label

The label on cleaners usually tells you the materials on which the product works best: floors, glass, tile, laundry, etc. All-purpose cleaners work on a variety of materials. Cleaners do not, however, mention any ability to remove microbes because a product must be tested according to government requirements before it can claim it kills germs. Although cleaners undoubtedly remove many microbes from hard surfaces or fabrics, the lack of testing means you cannot be sure of exactly how well they remove microbes.

Disinfectants

A disinfectant is a chemical solution that kills all microbes except bacterial spores on hard, inanimate surfaces. (*Bacillus* and *Clostridium* are two bacteria that make endospores, also called spores.) In other words, this is the most effective product you can buy to kill any germs thought to be lurking in your kitchen, bathroom, office, etc.

Disinfectants are registered with the Environmental Protection Agency (EPA) so that you can be assured they fulfill the claims printed on their label. Disinfectants must list by name the microbes they kill and they must include directions for use. Only by following the directions for use can you be sure you are killing germs.

How do microbiologists test disinfectants against all of the world's microbes? They cannot test the product against everything; if they did, a manufacturer would never get a chance to market its product. To pass the EPA's rules, microbiologists test disinfectants against one gram-positive microbe, represented by *Staph aureus*, and one gram-negative microbe, represented by *Salmonella*. (Products intended to be used in hospitals and other medical facilities must add a third test microbe, *Pseudomonas aeruginosa*.) In the disinfectant business, *S. aureus*, *Salmonella*, and sometimes *P. aeruginosa*, stand in for every other type of bacteria in the world.

Infection Vocabulary

Broad-spectrum and limited-spectrum disinfectants are two different types of disinfectants categorized by the variety of microbes they kill. A broad-spectrum disinfectant kills both gram-positive and gram-negative bacteria. In other words, this product gives you full coverage against diverse germs. A limited-spectrum disinfectant kills one or the other type of bacteria but not both. Limited-spectrum disinfectants are hardly ever sold because consumers have no way of knowing what type of germs they need to kill, and a limited product would not be a good choice in fighting infection.

Reading a Disinfectant's Label

Pick up a disinfectant in the cleaning aisle and read the label. Any product that has been tested and approved by the EPA to kill germs will, and must, have the following things on the label:

➤ The word *disinfectant* or *disinfects*

➤ The names of the microbes on which it has been tested

➤ The directions for use, including the number of minutes the product must be on the surface to kill the germs

➤ A list of ingredients

➤ An EPA registration number

Without these bits of information, you cannot be sure a cleaning product truly kills germs.

The Chemicals in Disinfectants

Are you worried about a cabinet full of disinfectants? Do you wish you didn't have to spray these products in the kitchen every day? Controversy swirls around the overuse of disinfectants and other products intended to kill germs, called antimicrobial products. Microbiologists have taken sides, with some believing we use too many disinfectants and others believing we don't use enough. In a pick-your-poison situation, the public must choose between chemicals or infection. Which would you rather have in your home? Everyone has a different opinion.

The chemicals in disinfectants are not strong poisons but neither are they harmless. Breathing their fumes can cause respiratory irritation and these products should not be put on the skin or the eyes. Pets are also sensitive to these products.

Before you become mired in an argument that has no resolution, consider doing the following. To reduce the chemicals used around your home, keep a disinfectant on hand but use it only when someone in the household is known to be sick or has a high risk of getting infection. (Review the high-risk groups mentioned in Chapter 2.) Use the product on the frequently touched surfaces that have the highest likelihood of carrying germs: countertops, faucet handles, refrigerator handles, flush handles, and toys if children are present.

Microbe Basics

Green products are intended to be safer than strong chemicals for the environment. This is usually true, but eco-friendly cleaning products seldom meet the EPA's requirements for killing germs. That is why you will not see the words *disinfect* or *sanitize* on green products.

Homemade cleaners can kill some germs but usually not as quickly or effectively as the strong chemicals that have been registered with the EPA. Solutions of white vinegar, lemon juice, and baking soda inhibit germs a bit but are not adequate protections against colds, flu, food-borne pathogens, or harder-to-kill pathogens like TB.

Sanitizers

Sanitizers are similar to disinfectants but instead of killing all microbes, sanitizers merely reduce the number to safer levels. They do this by containing weaker chemicals than those found in disinfectants or by requiring less time to work.

Disinfectants can take as long as ten minutes to kill the microbes on your kitchen countertop; a sanitizer might need only one minute, a definite advantage. The term for this waiting period is *contact time*. Most people will not wait the entire ten minutes a disinfectant requires before wiping the surface dry. People are more likely to follow a product's directions if they must wait only sixty seconds, or sometimes only thirty seconds, to kill germs.

A disadvantage of sanitizers lies in the mysterious claim, "reduces germs to safe levels." Do we really know what a safe level of pathogens might be? The people who make sanitizers have no idea if your household is home to an elderly person, a chemotherapy patient, or a cancer survivor. You have no idea if you're trying to kill *Salmonella*, 1,000 cells of which are needed to start infection, or *Shigella*, 10 cells of which can make you sick.

Infection Vocabulary

Health care professionals refer to disinfectants with terminology that is different from what I present here. Though the words differ, the meanings stay the same. In their terminology, a high-level disinfectant is a chemical that sterilizes a surface. An intermediate-level disinfectant is equivalent to a disinfectant, and a low-level disinfectant equals a limited-spectrum disinfectant.

Reading a Sanitizer's Label

Sanitizers must tell you the percent by which they reduce germs. A claim of killing 99.9 percent of bacteria in sixty seconds means that if 1,000 microbes are on your bathroom counter, only one will remain after using this product. But if you spill hamburger juices in the kitchen, you might be looking at a million bacteria on the countertop. Reducing this microbial load by 99.9 percent still leaves 1,000 bacteria behind. That's enough to make you sick.

"How about if I just leave the sanitizer on a little longer to kill more things?" I get this question often. Leaving the sanitizer on longer provides a little more killing action, but it will probably never be as effective as a disinfectant. (Some manufacturers make formulas that work as both a disinfectant and a sanitizer. To sanitize, you leave it on the surface for a minute or so and to disinfect, you let it work the full ten minutes.)

The EPA controls the testing and sale of sanitizers, too. Sanitizers must have the same things on the label as disinfectants, except they instead include the word *sanitizer* or *sanitizes*.

Microbe Basics

The various types of infectious agents differ by how hard they are to kill. This is why following the label instructions is important. A contact time of ten minutes really means ten minutes if you want to kill the germs listed on the product's container.

The following microbes are listed in order from the hardest to kill to the easiest:

➤ Bacterial spores (*Bacillus, Clostridium*)

➤ TB bacteria

➤ Viruses without lipid coats (cold virus, polio)

➤ Fungi (athlete's foot, *Candida* yeast)

➤ Bacteria (*Salmonella, E. coli, Staphylococcus*)

➤ Viruses with lipid coats (hepatitis, HIV, cytomegalovirus)

Prions are the most resistant infectious agents of all.

Kitchen Germs and Bathroom Germs

The cleaning aisle offers an impressive array of specialty products. Want to kill only bathroom germs? No problem, because Company X has a bathroom disinfectant just for you. Are kitchen germs keeping you up at night? Buy Company Y's kitchen sanitizer. Company Z has just started advertising its food surface sanitizer, so you can really home in on a specific place in your kitchen. Can a product for disinfecting the refrigerator door handle and another for disinfecting the dishwasher door handle be far behind?

Germs don't read the labels. Sure, you should expect to find more fecal microbes like *E. coli* in the bathroom than in the kitchen. But germs get around. The kitchen has tons of *E. coli* and other fecal microbes that come in on your hands, with kids and pets, and on groceries. There is no need to buy a dozen different antimicrobial products when all you need is one.

Microbe Basics

The term *superbug* refers to any microbe that resists the action of either antibiotics or chemical disinfectants. Many antibiotic-resistant bacteria have evolved since the commercialization of antibiotic drugs. Resistant superbugs have become a major health threat because fewer drugs are now available to fight infection.

More microbiologists are starting to believe that a new generation of bacteria resistant to chemical disinfectants may also soon emerge. This they surmise will happen because of the overuse of chemical cleaners in the home just as antibiotics were overprescribed for decades. Lab experiments have shown that the mechanisms used by bacterial cells to resist antibiotics may also resist chemicals.

The jury is still out on whether we are developing new chemical superbugs, but the history of antibiotic use does not give comfort.

Using Germ-Killing Devices at Home

Microbiologists use lamps that emit ultraviolet (UV) light to kill contaminants inside laboratories and to remove potential pathogens from water. Now, the idea of zapping pathogens with UV has moved into the home, too. Some brands of vacuum cleaners contain a small UV lamp. As the vacuum sucks up dust and dirt, the tiny particles are exposed to a brief flash of UV light. Does it work to kill germs?

UV light damages the DNA inside every living cell. In higher organisms, this represents a potential cause of cancer. In prokaryotes, the exposure means death. Bacteria cannot grow if they cannot replicate. If their DNA has been damaged seriously enough by exposure to UV, they reproduce no more.

Small UV exposures of vacuumed dirt will probably not kill all the microbes zooming through your vacuum hose. For one thing, the microbes can hide inside large chunks of dirt and escape exposure altogether. Second, the exposure time is probably not sufficient to kill all the microbes in heavy dirt loads. Finally, bacteria have a repair kit inside their cells. If their DNA sustains minor nicks from UV light, enzymes repair the damage. As usual, the resourcefulness of microbes puts human technology to shame!

Some vacuum cleaners also tout a special filter called HEPA, which stands for "high-efficiency particulate filter." HEPA filters are very good at taking tiny dust and other particles, even viruses, from the air. Places that require the cleanest conditions possible install HEPA filters in their ventilation systems to remove all possible contaminants. Thus, operating rooms, manufacturing plants that make computer chips, and facilities that produce injectable drugs rely on HEPA filters to keep their surroundings free of airborne contaminants.

Do you need a HEPA filter or a UV light in your vacuum cleaner? Both devices aim to remove microbes from the air that escapes from a running vacuum cleaner. Vacuuming stirs up a lot of particles and the principle behind HEPA filtration or UV exposure seems valid. Overall, these additions to your cleaning probably remove few microbes compared to the enormous numbers coming into your home with foot traffic, on clothing and pets, and on the breeze.

Try not to overdo home cleaning to the point where you think germs are everywhere. They *are* everywhere, but you need not sterilize your world to be healthy. We can live in peaceful coexistence with most germs.

Tips on Reducing the Germs You Meet

Spend a day with a germophobe or a microbiologist. Your experience might be enlightening as you see the world through the eyes of someone who "sees" germs everywhere.

Your bathroom and kitchen surfaces likely contain more microbes than any other place in your home. The only places that rival the bathroom and kitchen are young children's rooms and pet areas. Bacteria outnumber all other germs here, but fungal spores can be prevalent, too, especially in seasons when windows are open. Virus numbers should be low unless someone in the house has a viral infection affecting the respiratory tract. You know what to do: keep surfaces clean and use a disinfectant if you're worried that fecal microbes are lurking. Don't forget that foods you bring into the home might be sources of fecal microbes also.

On the way to work, note the surfaces you share with strangers. The buttons on ATM machines, the handle on the creamer at the coffee shop, grips and straps, gas pumps, railings and doorknobs and levers—the list goes on. You could pull out a can of disinfectant to spray all these places, but the can would be empty by the time you made it to work. Better to be mindful of those surfaces and wash your hands as soon as possible once you arrive at work. Don't touch your face or any food that you hold directly (bagels, doughnuts, fruit, etc.) until you have washed your hands or at least used an alcohol-based hand sanitizer.

Shaking hands does you no favor either, but by convention we do this simple act as a sign of friendship. Whipping out a hand sanitizer immediately afterward may please a germophobe but insult your colleagues. The rules of good hygiene begin with your hands. By paying attention to the things you touch, you can block germ transmission more effectively than depending on the strongest disinfectants.

CHAPTER 13

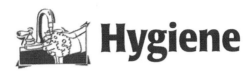 # Hygiene

---

In This Chapter

➤ Two different types of hygiene and how they promote good health

➤ How to wash hands to remove germs

➤ The basics of personal hygiene and oral hygiene

➤ Tips on removing germs from laundry

In this chapter you will learn tactics for good personal hygiene. Even if germs cover every surface around you and each person you meet is a potential carrier of infection, you can fight infections by following basic principles of good hygiene. You can't control the germs that others may carry, but you can prevent these germs from harming you as soon as they come in contact with your body. That is the goal of hygiene.

Beware: hygiene is difficult to assess in others. Lots of us think our own personal hygiene is top-drawer but suspect the hygiene of others to be woefully substandard. But messiness, slovenliness, or disorganization are not necessarily signs that a person has poor personal hygiene habits.

Hygiene is a process for preserving health and it applies to communities as well as to individuals. Community hygiene involves all the measures taken at the local, state, and national levels to control communicable diseases. Personal hygiene involves the steps taken by you to prevent getting infected by the pathogens that cause these diseases.

Hygiene Always Starts with the Hands

I refer often to good hand-washing techniques because they are critical to blocking the spread of germs. It's time to take a closer look at hand washing.

Hand washing removes dirt that may carry pathogens as well as transient microbes. Transients are the microbes picked up by your skin from other people, plants, animals, and inanimate objects. These microbes rarely establish a permanent residence on your skin because your normal flora prevents it. Transients present a risk of opportunistic infections when you have a break in the skin due to injury or burn or your immune system is severely weakened.

To rid the hands of dirt and transients, which have the potential to include a pathogen or two, wash your hands in the following circumstances:

➤ After using a restroom

➤ After sneezing or coughing (assuming you've covered your mouth and nose with your hand)

➤ Before eating or preparing meals

➤ After touching raw meats and fish

➤ After touching pets or livestock

➤ After handling animal products such as hides or pelts

➤ After being on an airplane

➤ After diapering a baby

Since infants and young children collect germs like Velcro, consider washing your hands after every time spent with them. In fact, any time you are dirty or sense that you've been around germs (think sporting events, public transportation, zoos, the grocery store shopping cart, etc.), wash your hands.

The proper way to wash your hands goes like this:

➤ Use soap and warm running water; avoid very hot water.

➤ Scrub all parts of the hands, including between the fingers and the fingertips.

➤ Continue washing for twenty to thirty seconds or while singing "Happy Birthday to You" twice.

➤ Dry all parts of the hands thoroughly to prevent chapping

Other tips for washing hands include using paper towels rather than a shared cloth towel and using liquid soaps dispensed by a pump rather than bar soap. Microbiologists have done studies on bar soaps that show bacteria accumulate on the soap's surface.

When you know you should wash your hands but no sink or restroom is available, carrying a small bottle of alcohol-based hand sanitizer serves as a good backup. Alcohol dries skin, leading to cracking (a portal of entry for pathogens), so don't rely solely on alcohol sanitizers.

Microbe Basics

Antimicrobial soaps went from being a terrific invention for fighting infection when first introduced to a cause for alarm by those wondering if they lead to resistant superbugs. Microbiologists no longer recommend the use of antimicrobial soaps for two reasons: the active chemical may be promoting the development of chemical-resistant microbes, and the chemical requires a contact time that few people will achieve.

Personal Hygiene

What goes into a good personal hygiene regimen? Hand washing, showering, and good dental care are obvious parts of personal hygiene. Personal hygiene also includes your immediate sphere, that is, the things you come in contact with daily. By extending cleanliness outward from your body to your personal space, you can reduce the chance of infection.

Here are some things to consider as part of your personal hygiene:

➤ Regular laundering of clothes and bedding

➤ Changing the bathroom towels every few days

➤ Wearing shoes and sandals and, especially in the case of sandals, washing your feet before bed

➤ Keeping children and pets clean

➤ Keeping your kitchen and bathroom looking clean

➤ Vacuum and dust inside your home

➤ Remove food, wrappers, and other trash from your car, and occasionally clean the interior of your car

➤ Remove garbage

> ➤ Regularly clean out the refrigerator and freezer

Hygiene never used to be taught in schools. Parents told their kids to cover up before sneezing and coughing. They kept sick children home from school. They preached the dos and don'ts of sharing. Somehow, the message of hygiene got lost. I see adults do things with their bodies that once upon a time only a four-year-old would do. Fortunately, the word is spreading again that people should take responsibility for preventing infection in themselves and should take steps to keep it from spreading to others.

Watch Out for the Hygiene of Others

If you see an adult doing something that clearly poses a threat to his or her health or yours, it's okay to speak up. Be prepared, however, to be rebuked. Criticizing someone else's personal hygiene is risky. Here are some of the things I've personally seen. What would you do if you saw these activities?

> ➤ A food vendor fished around in her mouth, picked something out of her teeth, and then without washing or wearing gloves plunged her hands into a salad mix to be served to paying customers.
>
> ➤ A waiter, standing next to the restaurant's kitchen door, picked his nose while waiting for his order.
>
> ➤ A woman on a flight diapered her baby on the empty seat next to hers.
>
> ➤ A man in a movie theater let loose a violent sneeze without covering up, spraying half a dozen people in the row ahead of him.
>
> ➤ A child in a restaurant was running between tables and stopped to cough right next to a table where meals had just been served.
>
> ➤ A coworker decided which bagel to select in the staff meeting by touching each and every one with his fingers.

I spoke up in about half of the instances described here. My diplomatic tries at explaining the importance of hygiene earned a very undiplomatic response. Perhaps even more demoralizing is that this is only a small sample of the many instances of hygiene disasters I've seen.

Oral Hygiene

Maintaining oral, or dental, hygiene is part of a good personal hygiene regimen. The mouth is a major thoroughfare for infectious agents. These microbes cause tooth cavities, gum and periodontal disease, respiratory infections, or gastrointestinal infections. Good oral hygiene keeps some of the trouble at bay.

The following activities make up good oral hygiene:

➤ Regular brushing, morning and evening or after meals, over the surface of the teeth and between the teeth

➤ Brushing the tongue from the front of the tongue to the back

➤ Regular use of floss on all teeth

Infections and Disease

Microbiologists appear on television morning shows to talk about the newest germ hot spots they have discovered. Because of this public service, many people now realize that an airplane's interior contains surfaces that hold millions of bacteria, fungi, and viruses.

Security screening has added a new germ hot spot. Passengers who go barefoot through security risk getting athlete's foot and more serious infections if they have a cut on their foot. Some airports lay down chemically treated rugs to prevent foot infections, but with many thousands of passengers tramping on the rugs every day, they probably don't kill many germs. The security pat down has also been implicated as a way to transmit germs from one person to the next.

It's hard to adhere to the best principles of hygiene in air terminals and airplanes. Do your best to reduce the risks by wearing socks, carrying hand sanitizer, avoiding as many shared items as possible, washing hands after the flight—and stop touching your face!

➤ Removal of impacted food debris

➤ Plaque removal by a dental hygienist or dentist at least twice a year

Unlike other parts of western medicine, dental care is primarily preventive. Listen to your dentist's recommendations. An unhealthy oral cavity affects your overall health, nutrition, and social life.

The Hygiene Hypothesis

The hygiene hypothesis is a theory developed in 1989 by pediatrician Erika von Mutius stating that regular exposure to microbes is good for our immunity and health. This theory appears in few textbooks and several eminent microbiologists have dismissed it as hogwash.

There is nonetheless a common ground that we must establish with the microbes in our environment. Perhaps being "too clean" does not benefit us.

From birth, an animal is exposed to microbes from its mother, then other family members, and then the surroundings. This early exposure to germs helps the immune system develop. Animals that scientists have raised in germ-free conditions have a hard time maturing into healthy adults. Their immune system and digestion never fully mature and these animals often die young.

Proving how microbes strengthen a developing immune system is not as easy as showing that exercise strengthens muscles and bones. Furthermore, it is hard to control the type of microbes to which a child is exposed. The hygiene hypothesis seems silly if we are facing a typhoid or plague epidemic.

Personal hygiene involves a rational approach to cleanliness and germ fighting. Common sense plays a big part. Most people intuitively know that six showers a day is excessive but taking only one shower a month is not enough.

Personal hygiene should be vigorous enough to keep you in the normal range of health relative to the community where you live. This means getting one to three colds a year, a case of the flu about every three to four years, an occasional food-borne illness, and perhaps one or two severe infectious diseases in a lifetime.

Microbe Basics

Household bleach is a chlorine-containing solution called sodium hypochlorite. Bleach is a very strong oxidizer, which is a chemical that destroys biological membranes and enzymes—one of the reasons why it removes stains. As such, it is one of the most effective disinfectants you can buy.

Because bleach is such a strong chemical, some myths have grown around it. One myth is that bleach is a good cleaner. It's not because it contains no detergent. Cleaning requires a detergent to remove the greases that hold dirt to hard surfaces. Another myth is that bleach is a poison. It's not. Chlorine gas is a poison, but bleach turns into water and salt when it degrades. Still another myth is that bleach is harmful to the environment. It's really less harmful to the environment than most other strong chemicals.

Germs in the Laundry

You wash your hands, cover up when sneezing, avoid the fellow coughing nearby. In other words, you follow all the principles concerned with fighting infection. It's laundry day. Now you separate darks, whites, and light colors and head for the washing machine. In the first load, in go the dish towels, washcloth, socks, and underwear. You have just contaminated a load of laundry with nasty fecal microbes.

Contrary to popular belief, a wash cycle does not kill germs. This is especially true since people today prefer to use cold water washes to save energy. All a washing machine does is make microbe soup. Fortunately, there are tips to reducing the spread of germs on laundry day:

> ➤ A name-brand detergent in an orange bottle is pretty good at killing bacteria.

> ➤ Hot-water washes reduce microbial numbers better than cold washes.

> ➤ A few products are sold that claim to sanitize laundry.

> ➤ For white loads, bleach is an excellent laundry sanitizer.

> ➤ Using a dryer for more than fifteen minutes effectively kills many germs.

A Word about Community Hygiene

Your community's hygiene program indirectly protects you against infection. By ensuring a clean living and working environment, a town lifts the overall health of its residents. To assess your community's hygiene program, look for the following:

> ➤ A water utility that offers open houses and provides residents with regular written reports on the community's water quality

> ➤ Good drinking water and sewer infrastructure without leaks and capable of handling overflows during heavy storms

> ➤ Infrastructure for wastewater and rain runoff

> ➤ Regular trash pickup

> ➤ Waste-recycling programs to reduce landfill burden

> ➤ Insect vector-control programs

> ➤ Animal-control and animal-vaccination programs

> ➤ Food inspections at restaurants and open-air markets

As with people, you can tell a lot about a community's hygiene just by observing.

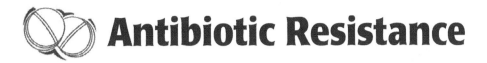# Antibiotic Resistance

In This Chapter

> Antibiotics and types of antimicrobial drugs

> Describing the ways to classify antibiotics

> The main antibiotic groups in use today

> Details on the way antibiotics kill bacteria

> Mechanisms of antibiotic resistance in bacteria

> Mistakes people make when taking antibiotics

> The problem of antibiotics in animal feed

In this chapter we explore the important subject of microbial resistance to antibiotics. Antibiotics are the final defense after an infection slips past your first-, second-, and third-line defenses. What if antibiotics fail to stop infection? This question has become a growing concern in medicine as doctors discover more antibiotic-resistant microbes in their patients.

In the two decades following the introduction of antibiotics, which was in the 1940s, these drugs seemed to be miracle cures for everything. Public health officials predicted the end of infectious disease. But by the 1960s, doctors found that a few infections once cured by penicillin seemed to be persisting. By switching to another antibiotic, the doctor could get the infection to go away. Before long, though, the second antibiotic seemed less effective. By the 1990s, antibiotic resistance in pathogens appeared to be the rule rather than the exception. Few of the antibiotics first introduced in the 1940s and 1950s are still in use.

This chapter introduces you to the names of antibiotics you are most likely to hear. It then explores the subject of antibiotic resistance and talks about the main resistant microbes that currently threaten our health the most. Because doctors now have a dwindling list of drugs for fighting infections, your dedication to personal hygiene, proper use of disinfectants, and blocking germ transmission become all the more crucial.

What Are Antibiotics?

The word *antibiotic* translates to "against life." Thus, antibiotics are substances that inhibit living things. Microbiologists reserve the term *antibiotic*, however, for a drug that kills only bacteria. Antibiotics do not kill viruses, so they are useless against colds and flu.

Microbiologists use the following terms for drugs that target specific types of microbes:

➤ Antibiotic: A drug that inhibits or kills bacteria

➤ Antiviral: A drug that inactivates viruses

➤ Antifungal: A drug that inhibits or kills fungi, including yeasts

➤ Antiprotozoal: A drug that inhibits or kills protozoa

Antibiotics are made by fungi and bacteria to kill unrelated species of bacteria. These substances work outside the microbial cell at very low concentrations. Antibiotics serve microbes in nature by eliminating competition from other microbes for nutrients and space.

No single antibiotic kills every known microbe. Antibiotics target specific pathogens or groups of pathogens. Doctors choose between two types of antibiotics when treating a patient's infection:

➤ Broad-spectrum antibiotic: Inhibits a large number of pathogens. These antibiotics are used when the doctor is not sure of the cause of infection or if more than one pathogen is causing infection.

➤ Narrow-spectrum antibiotic: Inhibits a limited number of pathogens. These antibiotics are used when the doctor knows the cause of infection.

Antibiotics fit into categories based on where they have been made. Natural antibiotics come directly from an antibiotic-producing microbe. Synthetic antibiotics are made in a laboratory by a chemist. Semisynthetic antibiotics have a component from the natural compound and a component that was synthesized by a chemist.

Infections in History

British chemist Alexander Fleming stumbled on the discovery of penicillin almost by mistake in 1928. He had left out on his lab bench some *Staphylococcus* cultures. When after a few days he returned, he noticed mold growing on the cultures. In the spots where the mold grew, no bacteria could grow. With a few experiments, Fleming showed that a substance excreted by the mold could kill bacteria.

Penicillin

Penicillin is naturally made by the fungus *Penicillium*. It kills bacteria by interfering with their ability to build a strong cell wall. Penicillin-treated cells become weak and cannot withstand physical stresses in their environment.

The mass production of penicillin began during World War II and continued unabated. With the rise of this and other antibiotics came a rise in penicillin-resistant bacteria. *S. aureus* contains an enzyme that efficiently snips penicillin apart whenever the bacteria see it. Today's versions of penicillin contain molecules that try to confound the bacteria, but it has been hard to stay ahead of the exquisite adaptability of these microbes.

Penicillin was indeed a miracle drug. It saved so many lives for the Allies in World War II that it has been credited as a major reason for the war's end. Penicillin has similarly saved lives that used to be lost to scarlet fever, rheumatic fever, and staph infections. The search for a more effective antibiotic has been daunting, but penicillin-resistance has made this task crucial.

How Antibiotics Work

Antibiotics are such a diverse group of compounds that microbiologists have put them into groups based on how they destroy bacteria. A bacterial cell is simple, but it has plenty of places that if damaged can stop the microbe's growth. Following are the various ways different antibiotics stop a pathogen's growth:

➤ Disrupt cell wall synthesis

➤ Inhibit protein synthesis

➤ Inhibit DNA synthesis

➤ Injure membranes

➤ Block key steps in nutrient metabolism

The manner by which a drug works in the body is called its mode of action. Antibiotics' mode of action against infection is to kill the infectious agent. The activities against bacteria listed above can also be thought of as the mode of action. For example, penicillin's mode of action against *S. aureus* is to disrupt cell wall synthesis so that new staph cells lack this critical protective layer and die.

Microbe Basics

Beta-lactam antibiotics consist of all antibiotics with a chemical structure called a beta-lactam ring. Many bacteria that resist these antibiotics do so by releasing an enzyme to destroy the ring. Without an intact beta-lactam ring, the antibiotic loses its effectiveness. Any bacteria said to possess the enzyme beta-lactamase or penicillinase are resistant to these antibiotics.

Some beta-lactam antibiotics are the penicillins, cephalosporins, cephamycins, and carbapenems.

The Main Antibiotics

Microbiologists categorize antibiotics in more than one way. As you've seen, antibiotics belong to different categories based on their spectrum of activity, their source, and their mode of action. Another way to classify exists based on the antibiotic's chemical structure.

I give the details of this type of grouping for two reasons: it is the most common way doctors and microbiologists talk about antibiotics, and grouping by antibiotic structure also relates to how bacteria resist the antibiotics. Here are the main antibiotic groups:

➤ Penicillins: Contain nitrogen and a component called a beta-lactam ring; work best against gram-positive bacteria. Examples are penicillin, ampicillin, methicillin, and oxacillin.

➤ Tetracyclines: Contain chlorine; have broad-spectrum activity. Examples are tetracycline, chlortetracycline, and oxytetracycline.

➤ Cephalosporins: Similar to penicillins. Examples are cephalothin, cefoxitin, and cefixime.

➤ Sulfonamides or sulfa drugs: Contain sulfur, have broad-spectrum activity, and even affect some protozoa. Examples are sulfamethoxazole, sulfadiazine, and sulfathiazole.

➤ Aminoglycosides: Contain an amino acid and are usually more effective against gram-negative bacteria. Examples are gentamicin, kanamycin, streptomycin, and neomycin.

➤ Quinolones: New versions (fluoroquinolones) contain fluorine and are widely used for UTIs, gastrointestinal infections, respiratory infections, and STDs. Examples are ciprofloxacin and ofloxacin.

➤ Macrolides: Made up of three antibiotic components, these have broad-spectrum activity. Examples are erythromycin and clindamycin.

Since biology has many exceptions, a few antibiotics fall outside these categories. Vancomycin and chloramphenicol do not fit into any of the above groups. Vancomycin acts similarly to penicillin and became an alternate treatment against infection when pathogens started becoming resistant to penicillin. Chloramphenicol is weaker than most other antibiotics so is prescribed in high doses. The high doses can cause side effects, so doctors prescribe this drug only when all others have failed.

How Bacteria Resist Antibiotics

Resistance is the ability of bacteria to live in the presence of an antibiotic meant to kill them. Susceptibility is the opposite; it is vulnerability to an antibiotic.

Bacteria have not been on Earth for 3.5 billion years without developing clever adaptations for their survival. Antibiotic resistance came in handy when bacteria encroached in the territory of an antibiotic-producing fungus. Then humans came on the scene and eventually stumbled onto antibiotics as a much-needed cure for infections. Antibiotic resistance became necessary for bacteria's survival.

Microbe Basics

Mutation is any permanent change in a cell's genetic material. It can happen in microbes as well as in humans and other higher organisms. Most mutations go undetected and have no effect on a cell's activity. Only when a mutation causes a change in the way a cell survives do we take note. In microbes, the mutations that give a species a greater ability to ignore the action of an antibiotic are the mutations that lead to resistance.

A mutated microbe enjoys an advantage over other members of its species that cannot resist antibiotic action. This explains why a mutation stays in a microbial population. Eventually, all members of the species retain the mutation that gives them a better chance at survival.

Resistance arises due to a mutation in bacteria's DNA. The mutation gives a cell an unusual ability to evade the antibiotic's action against it. When this resistant cell replicates, it sets in motion the development of a new generation of resistant cells. These are called resistant strains.

Resistant strains upend the antibiotic's action by any of the following mechanisms:

➤ Releasing an enzyme that destroys or deactivates the antibiotic

➤ Blocking the antibiotic's entry into the bacterial cell

➤ Ejecting the antibiotic from the cell as soon as it enters

➤ Using an alternate metabolism to bypass the antibiotic's action

Drug companies now try to invent new antibiotics that confound the bacteria's resistance mechanism. Of course, bacteria are the most adaptive organisms on Earth. They develop resistance to many of the new antibiotics in a short time.

Microbe Basics

During the early emergence of antibiotic-resistant pathogens, drug companies found success by making new versions of natural antibiotics. These were called next-generation antibiotics. For example, a chemist altered penicillin to make amoxicillin, then carbenicillin, cloxacillin, and so on. Each new version bought some time for doctors in treating infection. But some pathogens eventually developed resistance to the new version, too. Some antibiotics have passed their first and second generations and doctors now depend on third-generation drugs.

The Main Antibiotic-Resistant Bacteria

MRSA: The Staph aureus Superbug

MRSA stands for methicillin-resistant *Staphylococcus aureus* or *Staph aureus*. MRSA became the first medically important antibiotic-resistant pathogen. *Staph aureus* causes a variety of opportunistic infections, and the presence of MRSA makes each of these infections much more serious.

MRSA began developing when *Staph aureus* first became resistant to penicillin. Doctors switched to an alternate form of this antibiotic called methicillin, which worked for a while. In the 1990s, *Staph aureus* strains resistant to both penicillin and methicillin began showing up in hospitals. MRSA was soon declared a medical crisis in a number of health facilities.

Today, health care professionals confront an MRSA strain that resists all antibiotics in penicillin's class and also the cephalosporins.

MRSA infections have become so prevalent that they have been divided into two types:

➤ Healthcare-associated MRSA (HA-MRSA): Causes infections in people who have recently had surgery, were hospitalized, or spent time in other health care facilities. This is a major cause of nosocomial (hospital-related) infections.

➤ Community-associated MRSA (CA-MRSA): Causes infections in people who have not recently been in a hospital or other health care facility.

CA-MRSA shows up in almost any public place where many people share a facility or equipment. For instance, CA-MRSA can be prevalent in sports team training facilities, athletic clubs, swim clubs, daycare centers, and military bases.

Like regular staph infections, CA-MRSA causes fever, chills, skin abscesses, chest pain, headache, and muscle aches.

Doctors cannot guarantee that the current antibiotics used against MRSA will work for long. For now, they prescribe vancomycin. Other antibiotics that might work against MRSA infection are clindamycin, tetracycline, doxycycline, or linezolid.

VRE: Vancomycin-Resistant Enterococcus

VRE consists of various species of *Enterococcus*, an organism that lives in the intestines and sometimes on the skin. Like *Staph aureus*, *Enterococci* are part of your normal flora and do not normally cause infection. When VRE infect, they choose various portals of entry: the intestines, urinary tract, and skin wounds.

VRE has developed resistance against

Microbe Basics

A plasmid is a small piece of DNA that bacteria store in their cells separate from the main DNA. (This main DNA is called the chromosome.) Plasmids that carry genes for antibiotic resistance are called R factors or R plasmids.

Resistance spreads rapidly through bacterial populations because bacteria share plasmids. As they pass R factors among themselves, the resistance expands through a larger number of cells. These exchanges are not confined to a single species either; different species can exchange R factors and resistance.

several antibiotics and VRE infections can be particularly dangerous in hospitals, where other resistant microbes also threaten patient health.

VRE resists the same antibiotics resisted by MRSA, plus it resists vancomycin. Linezolid is the main treatment for infections.

Multiple Resistant Tuberculosis

TB has been called a reemerging disease in many parts of the world. This resurgence has happened because of human migrations to densely populated cities, global travel, and the development of drug-resistant TB strains. When infected people permanently move to new locations or travel across continents for short periods, they spread the TB pathogen.

TB is not an easy organism to kill in the best of circumstances. TB drug treatment takes a long time and requires four drugs. Perhaps because the drug regimen is hard to follow, patients may miss doses or stop treatment too early. These mistakes only add to the risk of developing a resistant pathogen.

Two resistant strains now threaten to make TB a worldwide problem. Both strains resist multiple antibiotics. The first is multidrug-resistant TB (MDR TB). MDR TB resists two of the four drugs needed to treat infection: rifampicin and isoniazid.

MDR TB has recently evolved into an even more resistant strain called extensively drug-resistant TB (XDR TB). XDR TB resists rifampicin and isoniazid as well as fluoroquinolone drugs that are part of modern TB therapy. XDR TB also resists some of the next-generation drugs that doctors have called upon to stay ahead of this pathogen's adaptability.

At present, people traveling to parts of the world where TB is a concern should seek information on XDR TB.

Mistakes We Make with Antibiotics

Forty years ago, doctors made the mistake of prescribing antibiotics for the wrong reasons. They dispensed antibiotics for virus infections, for unidentified illnesses, or simply because patients demanded them. They have learned from their mistakes and pay the price now by battling a growing list of resistant species.

To slow the emergence of new antibiotic-resistant bacteria, the rules for correct antibiotic use must be followed. Have you made any of the following mistakes? If so, I include reasons why these mistakes may lead to antibiotic resistance.

> ➤ Discontinuing your antibiotic treatment before the bottle is empty because you already feel better: This allows the stronger pathogens still remaining in your body to proliferate and possibly restart the infection.

➤ Taking the antibiotic when it is convenient rather than following the prescription's instructions: The drug should be present in the bloodstream in a constant amount to put continual pressure on the pathogens.

➤ Ignoring the prescription's instructions regarding taking the pill with food or drink: To work, the antibiotic must first be absorbed into the bloodstream. Drug companies have figured out the best conditions for absorption, so follow their instructions.

➤ Using expired drugs to save money: A weakened version of the antibiotic helps the pathogen resist it.

➤ Splitting pills to get more out of a prescription: A lowered level of antibiotic gives the pathogens more opportunity to build resistance.

The precautions you take against regular infections are the same for preventing infections by antibiotic-resistant microbes. Antibiotic-resistant bacteria come in contact with skin and mucous membranes the same way other bacteria do, and your body's defenses behave the same way toward them. Some resistant bacteria, such as MRSA, have a high degree of virulence. If your defenses don't hold their ground, antibiotic treatment becomes very important to your health. If the antibiotic cannot stop the infection, you're in trouble. This alone should give you added incentive to follow the principles of hygiene, cleanliness, and so on.

Antibiotics in Animal Feed

Many farms involved in meat, milk, or egg production include a small amount of antibiotics in the daily feed given to their animals. These drugs are given for two main reasons. One reason relates to the overcrowded housing that many animals endure in conventional farming and feedlots. Animals crowded close together and under stress can pass germs just as you pass germs during flu season when riding a crowded bus on the way to work. Farm owners feel the antibiotics help reduce the risk of infection in their animals. Another reason for antibiotic use in feed is the belief that the drugs improve the animals' performance. In other words, meat-producing animals grow faster when given antibiotics than they do without the drug. Getting cattle, pigs, or chickens to market faster means more money for the farm owner.

Farmyard antibiotics are given in subtherapeutic levels, meaning the drug is present in the animal's blood in levels too low to stop an infection. Despite the benefits antibiotics give to the business of agriculture, subtherapeutic levels also encourage the development of resistant bacteria on these farms. Microbiologists have now traced certain antibiotic-resistant pathogens from hamburger and other meat to farms that use antibiotics.

Antibiotic use on farms was once believed to be a sound decision for animal health and for farms. Now we know that this practice belongs on a long list of mistakes that people have made concerning antibiotics.

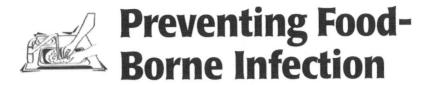

CHAPTER 15

Preventing Food-Borne Infection

In this chapter you will learn the principles of food-borne infections and how to prevent them. First, let's distinguish these infections from other bad things that can happen when you eat contaminated food.

Food-borne infections are caused by pathogens in food. Food poisoning, by contrast, comes from unwanted chemicals in food, such as the rat poison strychnine.

Food toxicities and food spoilage also result from microbes. A food toxicity occurs when microbes growing in food secrete a toxin that causes illness when eaten. Sometimes the microbes are no longer in the food, but the toxins remain, and they can make you sick. Food spoilage is caused by microbes that change the qualities of a food. Sometimes food spoilage microbes make food so unappealing that you don't want to eat it; other times, a spoilage organism can cause illness. This chapter will cover food spoilage because it can cause illness in some circumstances.

Humans have had a love-hate relationship with microbes in their food since ancient times. Early historical records give evidence that people have used bacteria and fungi to make certain foods for centuries. Bread, wine, and beer are some of our most ancient foods that need microbes.

Microbes transform foods, preserve food, and help digest food in our intestines. Microbes also spoil food or grow to enormous numbers so that a small bite can soon bring on gastrointestinal mayhem. The trick to maintaining good food quality and avoiding food-borne infection is to keep the good microbes in the foods where they belong and the bad microbes away from our meals.

Recognizing Food-Borne Infection

You cannot avoid food-borne infection. People make mistakes and sooner or later you'll eat a food that is contaminated. But knowing the characteristics of food-borne infections and the pathogens that cause them help reduce the incidence of these ailments.

The majority of food-borne infections you are likely to get in a lifetime have similar symptoms. These infections cause headache, fatigue, nausea, vomiting, fever, chills, and diarrhea. Most food-borne infections are acute: the symptoms appear quickly, the results are dramatic, and the illness goes away fast.

For these symptoms to occur, you must first ingest an infectious dose of a pathogen. Then the microbe must grow inside your body to numbers high enough to cause tissue damage or an illness-producing dose of toxin.

Most food-borne infections end without causing any permanent damage to your body. That's good news. The bad news is there will be no immunity to the pathogen and you will probably get another food-borne infection in your lifetime. Later in this chapter, I'll explain why the risk of food-borne infection may be increasing.

Epidemiologists recognize food-borne illness outbreaks by taking note of the classic symptoms listed above. Finding the source of most food-borne outbreaks can nevertheless be quite difficult. Not all infected people get the same symptoms in equal severity. Some people who eat the same tainted food manage to avoid ingesting an infectious dose or their immunity defends them. Outbreaks that start in restaurants are hard to trace because many diners may travel out of the area after eating there. Another reason these outbreaks are difficult to catch is that they tend to be underreported to doctors. Most people know they have eaten something that made them sick, but they also know the symptoms will probably subside. Life goes on. Only the biggest and most severe outbreaks make news.

Following are the signs of a food-borne outbreak in a community:

> ➤ Illnesses with similar symptoms clustered in the same neighborhood and in the same families

> ➤ Illnesses in many people who have recently eaten at the same location

> ➤ Increased absenteeism in a confined population such as military bases, campuses, cruise ships, convention centers, etc.

> ➤ Increased sales in diarrhea-control medicines and toilet paper

Why Microbes Grow in Food

Few things other than food provide the abundance of riches for a microbe's growth. High in nutrients and moisture, food is also stored at temperatures comfortable for microbial growth, and for periods of time that allow for many generations to reproduce. Since microbes have the same general nutrient requirements that people have, the most nutritious foods for us are also the foods most likely to have a pathogen growing in them.

Microbe Basics

Good restaurant hygiene includes evidence of cleanliness that extends from the front door to the wait staff, into the kitchen, and through the back door. Look for the following things to give you a sense of a well-run restaurant:

> ➤ Neat and manicured grounds and parking lot

> ➤ Clean and swept floors

> ➤ Clean tables and tablecloths

> ➤ Uniformed wait staff who are clean and well groomed

> ➤ No gum chewing among any of the staff

> ➤ Clean utensils and glassware

> ➤ An open, visible kitchen

> ➤ Rinsed salad greens

> ➤ Bussed tables

> ➤ Prompt and regular garbage removal from the kitchen

The microbes that grow well in certain foods have a constitution that matches the characteristics of a particular food. For example, molds that subsist in dry conditions do well in grains; lactobacilli, which like acidic conditions, grow well in acid foods. Let's look at how food microbiologists classify foods based on physical and chemical features of the food. Notice that some foods can belong to more than one category:

➤ High-moisture foods, such as fresh foods, salads, raw meat and poultry, pudding, soft cheeses, and eggs

➤ Low-moisture foods or foods in which water is chemically unavailable to the microbes, such as grains, nuts, cereals, crackers, sugar, uncooked pastas, jams and jellies, and honey

➤ High-acid foods (pH 1.8–5.3), such as citrus fruits, berries, tomatoes, mayonnaise, dry sausages, and breads

➤ Medium-acid foods (pH 5.4–6.6), such as most cheeses, peas, chicken and turkey, onions, corn, and egg yolks

➤ Low-acid foods (pH 6.7–9.5), such as cod, scallops, crab, and egg whites

➤ Microbe-inhibitory foods, which have natural antimicrobial components, such as acid foods, egg whites (contain lysozyme and other compounds that inhibit microbes), and spices (containing antimicrobial oils or extracts)

Infections and Disease

Summertime means picnics, grilling, and potato and macaroni salads. When a food-borne outbreak occurs, most people point to the mayonnaise. Dishes with mayo are associated with food-borne illness, but the mayo is not the problem. At a pH of about 4, mayo inhibits the growth of most microbes. But mayo is usually part of dishes that contain many different ingredients. Think chicken salad, macaroni salad, and potato salad.

Dishes with several ingredients increase a microbe's opportunities for nutrients, water, and hiding places. The hiding places may even protect microbes against the inhibitory effects of the mayo! These dishes are often held at warm temperatures for more than an hour, another invitation for microbial growth. Next time you feel queasy, don't blame the mayo.

Early societies learned that they could take advantage of a food's attributes to keep the food from spoiling. By drying food, freezing it, or adding things like sugar or salt to make water unavailable to microbes, the food held its nutrition but forestalled spoiling. Most of the preservative methods still used today have changed little from antiquity. The following methods all work because they make food a less hospitable place for microbes to thrive:

➤ Smoking and curing

➤ Salting

➤ Preserving with sugar or honey

➤ Fermenting to form acids

➤ Cooling and freezing

➤ Drying

The above preservation methods work by retarding microbial growth. Heating also makes food safer by killing the microbes, but heating (cooking) fails to guarantee a safe food. Microbes that have already grown to very high numbers in a precooked food may have released toxins into the food. The food industry uses all of the above methods plus chemical preservatives and radiation, both of which I'll discuss later.

The food industry strives to strike a balance between a preserved food that contains no pathogens and a palatable food that provides good nutrition. Plenty of foods could be made safe from contamination by loading them with so much salt, for instance, that no microbe would survive. But such a food would be next to impossible to eat. Few foods you eat are sterile. Food holds lots of microbes. Face it. The object of sound food preparation and preservation is to eliminate the pathogens from the food even if many innocuous microbes remain.

The Food Temperature Danger Zone

To reduce food-borne infection, do all you can to keep foods out of the temperature danger zone. Microbes grow fastest in a zone of about 40°F to 140°F. If you can't remember these exact temperatures or do not own a thermometer, remember the following:

➤ Refrigerate leftovers and groceries requiring refrigeration as soon as possible

➤ Cook foods immediately after preparation

➤ Cook foods above 150°F (above 240°F as a safety margin)

➤ Refrigerate and freeze foods in small containers rather than large containers (to speed the cooling)

➤ Thaw frozen foods in a refrigerator, not at room temperature

Do not allow any food to remain in the danger zone for more than two hours. The less time you give microbes a chance to multiply in foods, the better. This includes a sandwich you pack for work or the meal in your child's school lunch. A tuna salad sandwich may start off healthy when you prepare it at home in the morning, but that same sandwich will rise to room temperature during the ride to school and a morning spent in a locker.

To avoid illness from foods you know will be stored in the danger zone, alter the types of meals you prepare. Forget about tuna and chicken salads or processed meats in sandwiches.

Choose instead prepackaged but healthy foods. This includes individually packed tuna, cheeses, unpeeled or uncut fruits and vegetables, granola snacks, and bags of nuts.

Food-Borne Toxins

Chapter 5 acquainted you with toxins made by microbes. Many of these toxins are also food-borne. The food industry uses the term *food intoxication* to describe an illness caused by food-borne toxins. This is the same as a toxicosis.

The following are the main food-borne toxins:

> ➤ Shiga and shiga-like toxins: Made by various enteric (from the intestines) bacteria (*Shigella*, *E. coli*); causes diarrheal diseases

> ➤ Botulinum toxin: Made by *Clostridium botulinum*; prevalent in low-acid canned foods and home-preserved foods

> ➤ Perfringens toxin: Made by *Clostridium perfringens*, a common toxin in reheated meat dishes

> ➤ Bacillus enterotoxins: Made by *Bacillus cereus*; common in a range of medium- and low-acid reheated foods or foods with many ingredients (casseroles, salads, etc.)

> ➤ Staph enterotoxins: Made by *Staph aureus*; affects mainly processed meats, dairy products, and bread and bakery products

Toxins have no odor, they do not change the food's color or consistency, and they possess no flavor. For these reasons, you cannot count on cooking alone to make a food safe. Preventing contaminants is the key to avoiding any food-borne illness.

Food Spoilage

When food spoils it gives you a visual warning that something is amiss. Throughout history, preventing food spoilage was critical to a society's survival. When microbes proliferate in food, they use up the nutrients and produce wastes that drastically change the flavor, color, consistency, smell, and nutrition of food. A spoilage microbe may not necessarily be a deadly pathogen, but it causes its own set of risks to good nutrition.

Food manufacturers use the same methods for preventing spoilage as they use for preventing the entry of pathogens. That means smoking, salting, chemical preservation, etc.

Ancient societies lucked upon the discovery of some spoiled foods that still tasted good but resisted further spoilage. By letting select bacteria, yeasts, or fungi into certain foods—people in ancient societies had no idea of the exact microbes they used—the earliest microbiologists invented natural preservation. These so-called fermented foods remain today:

➤ Cheeses and yogurt from milk

➤ Breads from grains

➤ Beer and wine from grains and fruit juices

➤ Sauerkraut, kimchi, pickles, olives, and soy sauce from fresh vegetables and legumes

Infection Vocabulary

Pasteurization is a heat treatment for protecting certain beverages from spoilage microbes and pathogens. Milk and fruit juices are the most frequently pasteurized products—many states even require that milk be pasteurized to be sold in their state.

The pasteurization process is a combination of temperature and time that will kill microbes. Thus, the process can be an exposure of the beverage to 161°F for 15 seconds, 191°F for 1 second, or similar combinations. Pasteurization is a critical step for removing the TB pathogens *Mycobacterium bovis* and *M. tuberculosis* from raw milk.

The Food Distribution Chain

Food spoilage and the more serious food-borne infections and toxicities enter anywhere in the food distribution chain from the farm to your plate.

Many problems are prevented when food handlers pay attention to good personal hygiene. Food manufacturing companies also add a measure of insurance against contamination by sanitizing their equipment and sterilizing the food's packaging before filling. Food distributors use refrigerated trucks when the food needs to be kept cold. In labs, microbiologists check the food products for signs of contamination and hold back any suspect products.

Food distribution has a long list of hot spots where contamination can enter the food. By reviewing the news, you'll discover several food-borne outbreaks that have occurred in the past few years. In the cases where the cause was finally identified, notice the recurrence of certain hot spots, such as the following:

➤ Field workers who pick crops

➤ Fresh produce rinsing lines

➤ Field crops in the path of manure-contaminated runoff

➤ Cleaning and packing or canning facilities

➤ Slaughter facilities

➤ Trucking and warehousing

➤ Grocery stores and open air markets

➤ Restaurants and other food vendors

➤ Home preparation of meals

Keep an eye out for clues that a breakdown in the system occurred between getting the food from the farm to you. You will not catch every instance of contamination, but these clues help:

➤ Torn or broken packaging

➤ Bulging cans or leaking contents

➤ Visible dirt particles

➤ Off odors and colors

➤ Cold foods allowed to warm up or thaw

➤ Precut vegetables or fruits

➤ Deli-style dishes containing several ingredients and needing refrigeration

➤ Food handlers or preparers at restaurants, vendors, farmers markets or stands that are obviously not practicing good hygiene

Beware also of foods ordered through online catalogs. Expect these foods to arrive in perfect condition as you would expect a meal at a fine restaurant. Send back anything that looks suspicious. It helps to order only from established companies with a good track record of sending foods, including imported foods, through the mail.

The more you think about the food distribution chain, the more you'll uncover places where mistakes might happen.

Major Pathogens of Meat

Meat gets most of its contamination during the slaughter process, which has a high risk of spreading fecal microbes to the carcass. As a result, the main meat pathogens, other than *Listeria*, are fecal bacteria:

➤ *Campylobacter jejuni*: Found in pork, poultry, and beef

➤ *Salmonella*: Found in poultry and beef

➤ *Listeria monocytogenes*: Found in processed meats

➤ *E. coli*: Found in undercooked hamburger.

Microbe Basics

A prion is an infectious agent made from a single strand of protein. Prions cause disease in humans, livestock, and some wildlife by infecting the nervous system. The resulting diseases have different names depending on the species affected, but they are all similar. Thus prion infections in cattle lead to mad cow disease or bovine spongiform encephalopathy, infections in sheep and goats is called scrapie, and infections in humans goes by the names kuru, fatal familial insomnia, Creutzfeldt-Jakob disease, and Gerstmann-Sträussler-Scheinker syndrome.

All prion infections cause a fatal degeneration of brain tissue. On examination, the brain of infected individuals contains small pockets where the nerve tissue looks like it has disintegrated. The spongelike appearance gave rise to the term *spongiform encephalopathy*.

Different cuts of meats carry vastly different loads of bacteria. Ground meats are the worst because they have a large surface area per ounce of meat. This surface offers more room for microbes to attach, get nutrients and air, and multiply. Cuts such as steaks provide one relatively smooth surface. In steaks, the surface area per ounce is much smaller than that in hamburger. Have you noticed that most outbreaks associated with a meat product trace back to hamburger rather than steak?

Seafood receives contamination during a processing system similar to that of meat products. Seafood also has the hazard of being exposed to potentially contaminated waters. Some of the major pathogens of seafood are *Salmonella*, *Vibrio*, and *Plesiomonas*.

Major Pathogens of Dairy Products

Milk is very vulnerable to spoilage, so the dairy industry uses several precautions that require strict inspections by the government. Pasteurization, refrigeration, and irradiation are all common techniques used to protect dairy products.

The risk of contaminating milk is highest when cows are milked, during packaging, and during transfer to trucks. Important names in dairy product contamination are *Salmonella*, *Campylobacter*, *Listeria*, *E. coli*, *Shigella*, *Lactobacillus*, and *Yersinia*.

Microbe Basics

Food manufacturers sometimes kill any potential pathogens in food by irradiating it with gamma rays. Gamma irradiation can kill *E. coli*, *Staph aureus*, and *Campylobacter jejuni* in meat and other food products. In addition to meat, poultry, and dairy products, this method has been used for protecting spices, fruits, and vegetables.

Major Pathogens of Vegetables, Fruits, and Juices

Crops from commercial farms do not carry many microbes in the same way food animals carry microbes. The microbes that naturally live on plants do not pose a health risk to people. Plants can, however, be contaminated by microbes from the soil or in runoff. Rain and irrigation water carry fecal microbes from ranches, feedlots, and wildlife.

The newsworthy food-borne outbreaks from eating raw vegetables, fruits, or fruit juices almost always come from fecal microbes in water or feces. The sources of the fecal contamination is likely to be animals (domesticated or wild that walk through the growing fields) and humans.

Vegetables to be canned by commercial operations or in home kitchens sometimes carry the botulism pathogen. This type of contamination has become rare because of good sanitary practices, but it still happens sporadically and can be fatal.

Microbe Basics

Products for rinsing fresh vegetables and fruits at home have been tried in the past with little success. The rinse contains a mild bleach solution that might reduce the number of microbes clinging to the outside of foods. Consumers did not like the idea of putting a chemical onto the food, and food microbiologists doubted the usefulness of these products. For instance, the rinse does not remove microbes that are inside a vegetable's leaves or stalk. The rinsing technique was also inefficient and consumers failed to rinse many parts of the food.

Food Preservatives

The preservation of what we call processed foods uses a combination of heating and a chemical. Preservatives do not always kill microbes; they merely inhibit the microbes' growth. A preservative does not last forever and few foods can last an eternity. In fact, I would be suspicious of the nutritional value of any food that is still edible ten years after it was manufactured!

Infection Vocabulary

Processed foods are any food sold in a can or box or bought from the freezer section of the grocery store. Some bagged foods, such as salad mixes, are minimally processed.

Chemical preservatives allow these foods to be stored without spoiling for several months to a few years. Some chemicals are safe, familiar to us, and have been used for many years without causing any health side effects in people. The government puts these chemicals on the generally recognized as safe (GRAS) list. Sugar and salt are examples of GRAS list preservatives. Here are other preservatives on the GRAS list:

➤ Ascorbic acid

➤ Benzoic acid

➤ Butylated hydroxyanisole (BHA)

➤ Butylated hydroxytoluene (BHT)

➤ Methylparaben

➤ Propylparaben

➤ Propionic acid

➤ Sodium benzoate

➤ Sorbic acid

➤ Sulfur dioxide

The chemicals in the GRAS list are also used in cosmetics. Check some products from around your home and see how many of these chemicals you can find.

Microbe Basics

A high amount of salt or sugar in a food helps preserve it by keeping water away from microbes. Adding salt, sugar, or freeze-drying food lowers its water activity. The water activity scale ranges from 1.00 to 0.00. Sugar has a water activity of 0.10; some fresh fruits have an activity of 0.99.

Most bacteria require a water activity of at least 0.90. Fungi get by in slightly drier conditions with a value of about 0.85. Even so, it is clear that microbes cannot survive in very dry conditions.

CHAPTER 16

Preventing Waterborne Infection

In This Chapter

➤ The microbes normally found in drinking water

➤ How drinking water is treated

➤ How wastewater is made safe for the environment

➤ The main waterborne microbes causing infections

➤ The basics of water distribution systems and reservoirs

This chapter will introduce you to the main waterborne pathogens and how to avoid them. The symptoms and the pathogens that cause many waterborne infections resemble those of food-borne infections. But water gets contaminated in ways that differ from food contamination. Like food-borne infection, most waterborne infections are not fatal, but there are exceptions, so learning how to avoid all tainted waters is essential to good health.

Waterborne infections are a leading cause of illness and death worldwide. Though the water supply in the United States is safe in comparison to many other parts of the globe, waterborne outbreaks occur sporadically each year here. It pays to know how to avoid these infections at home and when you are traveling abroad.

What's in This Water?

All water you drink contains microbes. Tap water and bottled water can have as little as a few microbial cells to several hundred per glass. Viruses and bacteria are the most common contaminants in water. In the United States, protozoa and fungi are very rare in water but can be quite high in concentration in other countries.

The bacteria normally found in water do not harm you. Some proponents of the hygiene hypothesis believe these bacteria are essential for developing strong immunity in growing children. The goal of water treatment systems is to remove the pathogenic bacteria from water as well as the viruses, protozoa, fungal spores, and even helminthes (worms and larvae) that may be present at the water's source. Treatment systems also remove bacteria that sometimes occur in high numbers in surface waters that get a lot of sun. This means mainly photosynthetic *Cyanobacteria*.

Some communities also have a high amount of algae in their water source, usually a reservoir that gets good sunlight to promote algae growth. Algae and *Cyanobacteria* produce harmless compounds that give water an unpleasant or earthy odor and poor taste. The compound geosmin offers an example. The presence of off odors, flavors, or colors does not mean the water is unsafe. But these factors lead people to think the water is of poor quality, so treatment plants try their best to remove them.

A better sign of trouble relates to the turbidity or cloudiness of water. Cloudy water may indicate that the water contains tiny particles that slipped through the treatment plant's filters. As you learned from the chapter on airborne transmission, microbes love to attach to particles.

Microbe Basics

A boil water alert is a warning issued by a community's health agency to tell residents the water supply is not safe. Floods, hurricanes, and other natural disasters can overwhelm water and sewer infrastructures. As a consequence, the levels of pathogens rise in the water sources that supply a community with its clean drinking water.

When you hear your community has been so warned, boil all the water you plan on using for drinking, cooking, making ice, and brushing teeth. This includes water for pets. Treat the water for five minutes at a rolling boil. Some websites recommend only one minute of boiling, but this may not be sufficient to kill all pathogens.

Here are some other tips to follow in a boil water alert. Avoid using the dishwasher. You don't need to boil water, however, for bathing and when washing laundry.

How Drinking Water Is Treated

Drinking water treatment uses few high-technology methods. Most of water treatment involves settling, filtering, and even treatment with good bacteria that eat a lot of the organic matter dissolved in the water.

Very few water sources are pristine with no need for treatment at all. The cleanest water from deep wells usually runs through a filter of some sort before going to a tap. In the United States, our main sources for drinking water are reservoirs, lakes, rivers, and aquifers (underground pools or lakes).

The EPA oversees water treatment and sets regulations on the maximum amount of contaminants that can be in tap water. These contaminants are either chemical or microbial. The following typical water treatment system is set up to remove both kinds:

➤ Filtration: Removes particles, including microbes

➤ Flocculation: Adds chemicals that make little particles aggregate into bigger particles. This helps them settle out faster and take more microbes with them.

➤ Disinfection: Removes all the good bacteria plus any stragglers that are still in the water using chemicals, gas, or irradiation.

After disinfection, drinking water goes to distribution lines to your community. The result is clean tap water.

Microbe Basics

Chlorine is the most effective disinfectant in microbiology. It kills all infectious agents. Chlorine also kills the resistant spore form of *Bacillus* and *Clostridium*, providing the contact time is long, usually up to an hour.

Chlorine begins destroying every part of a microbial cell within seconds of contact. This chemical ruins membranes, stops the action of enzymes, and damages the structural compounds of the cell.

Chlorine dissipates in air so must be added regularly to bodies of water to maintain disinfectant activity. This includes pools, hot tubs, spas, and the water at recreational water parks.

Water Disinfection

Five types of water disinfection make drinking water safe. Chlorine treatment dominates the others in this country but things are changing. An increasing number of treatment plants are trying non-chlorine methods. Here are the ways these methods work:

> ➤ Chlorine compounds: Chlorine, chloramines, and chlorine dioxide gas each kill microbes quickly. The EPA wants treatment plants to put enough chlorine in water so that about 2 parts per million (ppm) remain as the water flows through distribution pipes. In reality, houses close to treatment plants get a bigger dose of chlorine than houses far from the plant. When you live at the end of the line, there is probably no chlorine at all in your water.

> ➤ Ozone: Exposing water to this gas kills microbes and doesn't have the chlorine odor and taste that consumers dislike.

> ➤ UV irradiation: This method exposes the water to UV light as water passes through pipes running between massive UV lamps. Cloudy water reduces the effectiveness of UV irradiation, and the lamps last only one to two years before needing to be replaced.

> ➤ Reverse osmosis (RO): This is the most effective way to remove the tiniest microbes. Water passes through very small pores in the filters, which trap microbes on the filter surface. Though this method is expensive, it avoids the use of chemicals and does not change water's taste or odor.

In-home water purification systems also use RO in combination with thick carbon filters that remove odor-causing compounds. If you use an in-home system, remember to change the carbon filter as directed. Microbes like carbon and view these filters as a big buffet table!

Water Distribution

When waterborne outbreaks occur, the problem may have started with a treatment plant using poor filters, inadequate settling and clarification steps, or faulty disinfection. Often, however, the problem begins after clean water has left the plant but before it reaches you.

Water distribution lines lie underground where they receive little maintenance or inspection. Some towns, such as New York City, rely on a century-old water infrastructure that somehow keeps millions of people safe from infection.

How do things go wrong underground? Here are some ways:

> ➤ Broken or corroded lines that allow soil microbes to pass into the distribution system

> ➤ Distribution lines situated too close to sewer lines, increasing the risk of cross-contamination if both lines break (think earthquakes)

> ➤ Outdated materials can be pitted even if the corrosion does not go all the way through the pipe. These pits help microbial colonies called biofilms to cling to the pipe interior. Biofilms grow to contain an enormous number of diverse microbes.

Water customers have little power to change the way their water is treated or comes to them. Some homeowners rely on in-home systems to add a little more oomph to the treatment process. Others resort to water delivery companies that supply bottled water. Beware of men in shorts bearing bottles! Bottled water can have several times more microbes than tap water, although they are seldom pathogens. Try not to store water in plastic bottles for long periods. Some bacteria in water get nutrients by eating the plastic.

Microbe Basics

Camping supply stores offer a variety of filtration devices for backcountry enthusiasts. These products work well in emergencies too. If you suspect the safety of your water has been compromised, use one of these pump style or pitcher style filtration devices.

Look for filters that use the words *absolute 1 µm*, which means all of the filter's pores measure no more than 1 micrometer in diameter. These filters remove all microbes larger than 1 micrometer from water. Filters that say *nominal 1 µm* have an average pore size of 1 micrometer. Some pores will be smaller than this size and others will be larger. Nominal filters, therefore, do not clean the water as well as absolute filters.

Keeping Reservoirs Safe

Reservoirs ideally lie in remote places outside of town. They are often at a higher altitude to save on costs of pumping water to homes. The remote location also helps the community's water utility keep the reservoir somewhat clean.

Reservoirs for drinking water should not allow swimming, wading, or similar contact between people and the water. Pets should not be allowed near reservoir water. In addition, boating isn't a good idea because of the fuel that enters the water. These precautions reduce the chance of humans', or Fido's, enteric microbes entering the water. Reservoirs still get exposure to wildlife and birds, both of which add microbes to the water. Even water from the cleanest-looking reservoirs need some treatment before you drink it.

Infections and Disease

The EPA sets standards for the maximum level of certain chemicals and microbes that are allowed in water. Good-quality water contains less than these allowable limits; poor-quality water misses the mark in one or more of EPA's criteria.

The EPA allows the presence of nonpathogenic bacteria in tap water. There should be no *E. coli*, viruses, protozoa, or microbial cysts present. The EPA also puts limits on water's turbidity, which helps ensure microbes cannot hide in small particles.

Major Waterborne Pathogens

Many of the main waterborne pathogens are also food-borne pathogens. Many food-borne infections come from foods that have touched contaminated water. Here are the microbes that treatment plants focus on for protecting your water supply:

➤ The bacteria *Aeromonas, Campylobacter, Helicobacter, Legionella, Leptospira, Mycobacterium, Pseudomonas, Vibrio*, and *Yersinia*

➤ The protozoa *Acanthamoeba, Cyclospora*, and *Naegleria*

➤ The protozoa-like cysts *Cryptosporidium* and *Giardia*

Not all of these microbes appear in all water supplies. In general, aquifers have fewer microbes than surface waters. Serious pathogens such as *Vibrio cholerae* and *Cryptosporidium* strike only in natural disasters, but they are both worth examining because of the severity of the diseases cholera and cryptosporidiosis, respectively.

Vibrio cholerae

Infections from *V. cholerae* have bothered society for centuries. Even today, outbreaks rage in areas affected by flooding, natural disasters, or a breakdown in water infrastructure. Some regions of the world have no safe water infrastructure at all. In these places, cholera is a constant menace.

Cholera is a severe acute disease that ravages the intestines. Without treatment, people can lose water from diarrhea, which leads to the collapse of the vascular system. Cholera claims thousands of lives worldwide each year.

The disease's incubation period ranges from a few hours to about five days. Symptoms are watery ricelike diarrhea that occurs in bouts, vomiting, muscle cramps, and extreme fatigue.

Treatments for cholera are limited to rehydration with intravenous fluids containing *electrolytes*. The quinolone antibiotics lessen the severity of cholera but do not completely eliminate the pathogen. No effective vaccine exists.

Travelers to countries where cholera is a risk should do the following things:

> ➤ Steer clear of water or ice made from water that hasn't been boiled.

> ➤ Say no to partially cooked or raw shellfish, uncooked vegetables, and fresh fruits

> ➤ Substitute fruits that must be peeled for unpeeled fruits and precut fruits.

> ➤ Swim only in chlorinated swimming pools

> ➤ Avoid ingesting water when washing or showering

> ➤ Brush teeth using bottled water

Doctors in regions with cholera are used to seeing this infection. Seek them out immediately if you suspect you have swallowed contaminated water.

Microbe Basics

Coliforms are a group of gram-negative bacteria common in natural waters, soil, on plants, and in an animal's intestines. Water treatment plants count the number of coliforms in water as an indication of possible contamination. But because coliforms can be found in so many places in nature, their presence in water does not automatically mean the water has been contaminated with dangerous microbes. For this reason, the EPA also requires local water utilities to monitor fecal coliforms. Fecal coliforms are known to come from animal or human intestines and make a better indicator of contamination. Some fecal coliforms are *E. coli*, *Klebsiella*, and *Enterobacter*.

For water to be considered safe and potable (drinkable), the EPA says it should contain no *E. coli*. The EPA does not set similar limits on coliforms and fecal coliforms, but it expects treatment plants to monitor for any trends and to react quickly if either type of bacteria begin to increase.

Cryptosporidium

Cryptosporidium is a protozoa-like microbe that forms a large cyst (6-8 μm diameter) that resists almost all heat and chemical treatments. Even the chlorine disinfection used in water treatment plants cannot kill all the cysts. Fortunately, the large size of the cyst makes it easier to remove from water than other microbes.

Cryptosporidiosis starts after ingesting ten or fewer *Cryptosporidium* cysts. The incubation period lasts four to fourteen days. Symptoms last from ten days to more than a month. Perhaps you are not surprised to learn that this infection is another characterized by severe diarrhea. In cryptosporidiosis, the diarrhea is accompanied by painful abdominal cramping.

The diarrhea occurs in waves between periods of relative calm. The periodic nature of the infection is due to the life cycle of the pathogen in the intestines as it reproduces and forms new generations of offspring.

In 1993, *Cryptosporidium* emerged as a pathogen to be reckoned with when it caused an outbreak in Milwaukee, Wisconsin, affecting 200,000 people. (The microbe had been discovered in 1976 but had not been connected with large outbreaks.) Health care providers deduced something was wrong when toilet paper and antidiarrheal medicines began flying off store shelves! The impetus for the contaminated water came from an unusually rainy period that overwhelmed wastewater treatment plants and led to spillover of untreated water into the drinking water supply.

The feces of infected people are extremely contagious, and cryptosporidiosis easily spreads to other family members. In case of infection, the best advice is to keep the sick individual isolated and supplied with his or her own towels, bedding, etc.

Little help exists for sufferers of cryptosporidiosis. Fluid replacement works best to alleviate harm to the body. The pathogen eventually leaves on its own.

Microbe Basics

Gray water is treated wastewater and sewage and the water that goes into shower drains and sinks. It's safe for the environment but not necessarily safe enough to be used for drinking and cooking. This water can have a higher number of microbes than clean drinking water and is much more likely to have pathogens. Some communities allow the use of gray water for irrigating agricultural fields.

Wastewater and Sewage

A fine line rests between wastewater and sewage. Wastewater consists of runoff from farms, neighborhoods, and storm drains. Sewage comes from the toilets and drains of houses and other buildings. Both accumulate the worst that humanity can produce!

Wastewater treatment plants play an underappreciated role in community hygiene. These plants clean up the waters flowing into them in about the same way that drinking water gets treated. Wastewater plants add a few steps, however, to remove the heavier loads of microbes, trash, and organic matter in wastewater and sewage:

➤ Filtration: The use of multiple filters in a wide range of pore sizes to remove everything from socks and medicine bottles to *Cryptosporidium* cysts.

➤ Aerobic digestion: The step in which a mixture of good bacteria is added to a tank. The mixture digests much of the organic matter from the water. By removing organic matter, the water becomes less delectable to microbes farther down the distribution line.

➤ Anaerobic digestion: The use of anaerobic bacteria in airtight tanks to digest the sludge that accumulates during the settling step. As an added benefit, these bacteria make methane gas as they work. Many treatment plants collect this natural gas and burn it for energy.

Disinfection occurs as the last step before the treatment plant releases the treated water back into the environment. As a final precaution in keeping this water away from you, treatment plants usually release the water offshore or into rivers where there are few people.

Infections and Disease

Stores selling outdoor and emergency supplies offer a variety of treatments for purifying water you suspect may be contaminated. (The word *purification* refers to the removal of anything unhealthy from water.) People can boil water or filter it through a water purification device. If these actions are not possible, try chlorine or iodine tablets.

For chlorine disinfection of water, add four drops of unscented household bleach that advertises 5.25 percent hypochlorite on the bottle to a quart of water. If you need a bigger volume, add sixteen drops (1/8 teaspoon) of bleach to a gallon of water, or 1 teaspoon of bleach to a 5-gallon bottle.

Iodine tablets are as effective as chlorine is on microbes and are easy to use. Follow the instructions on the package.

Warning Signs of Bad Water

Poor water quality is a problem on every continent, so water safety should be your first concern when traveling.

Cloudiness is the main visible sign of potentially tainted water. Other signs of trouble can be found in your surroundings. Check for the presence of garbage dumped in neighborhoods, rats scurrying at night, pets defecating in yards and streets, and laundry being taken to the nearby river. Societies that have only a local well as their water source are probably in a situation called water stress. Water stress occurs when a region's demand for clean water has outstripped the land's ability to supply it.

Few of us in the United States confront severe water stress like people do in more arid parts of the world. But water quality can decline quickly. During Hurricane Katrina, massive flooding contaminated all the water sources, and waterborne infection rapidly became the biggest threat to people's health.

PART FOUR

Fighting Infection

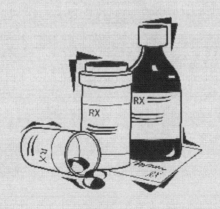

CHAPTER 17

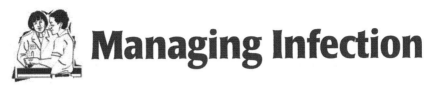

Managing Infection

In this chapter, you will consider the big picture of infection. The infection chain can be viewed from a personal perspective—how you get germs, what you do to fight the infection's symptoms, and how well you recover—as well as from a community perspective in which certain infections follow predictable patterns. This chapter will explain why taking a global view of infection might help you ward off infection on a personal level.

You will also revisit high-risk groups in this chapter, and get some tips on how to care for these individuals. Finally, this chapter tells you where to go for more information on infections, both rare and common.

Infection on a Global Scale

Infection follows certain patterns as it moves through societies. Without exception, the activities of a society determine who pathogens will infect in the population, how fast the infection will spread, and the length of time it will remain.

Following is a list of the factors in any region of the globe that influence the patterns of infection:

➤ Level of poverty and socioeconomic status

➤ Transportation infrastructure, which determines how fast people can reach medical care and how well medical supplies can be distributed

➤ Climate and weather, which affects the animals and insects that come in contact with people

➤ Geography, which determines plants, wildlife, weather, and extent of water stress

➤ Type of economy and occupation, which determines the germs people are exposed to; agricultural economies are exposed to germs different from those of service-based economies, and occupation affects the predominant types of transmission

➤ Genetics, which determines the susceptibility of the population

➤ National infrastructure, which determines the quality of water supply and sanitation systems

➤ Education

With these global considerations in mind, you might be able to add a few more. Think about all the ways that germ transmission and infection change over time.

Before 1980, no one had heard of AIDS. The disease would soon devastate segments of western society. At the same time as wealthier countries were increasing efforts to control the AIDS epidemic, poverty exploded in sub-Saharan Africa. A combination of politics, poverty, and faulty education led to an explosion of AIDS in a new part of the world and in different subpopulations: heterosexual men and women instead of homosexual men. AIDS didn't descend on humanity; it merely took the opportunity we gave it.

Infection control has two equally important pieces: infection prevention and infection treatment.

At the Doctor's Office

The One Health Initiative is a program supported by almost 1,000 scientists worldwide to coordinate the goal of fighting infection. It includes diverse human medical specialties, veterinarians, and dentists. The initiative may grow in importance as new zoonotic diseases emerge. By studying the relationships of environment, human health, and animal health, members hope to develop approaches to breaking the global infection chain.

Infection Control

Experts in global infectious disease take the same steps to solve the problem of infection as anyone looking at the problem from a personal perspective. They start with the pathogen, consider the host's susceptibility, examine possible transmission routes, and so on. Whether fighting infection in one person or in a large community, each link in the chain is equally important.

Take a look at the infection chain again, this time by thinking about where you fit in the issue of global infection:

➤ The pathogen: Some pathogens travel around the world (influenza) and others are confined to regions (Ebola virus). In your town, are you more likely to be exposed to the flu or Ebola? Do you work on a farm where the hay occasionally gets moldy or in an office building with mold in the walls?

➤ The pathogen's source or reservoir: Keeping an eye on potential reservoirs gives you important information on the likely infections coming your way. Do you live near a river or a desert? Does wildlife come into your yard at night? Do bats?

➤ Transmission: How do you guess most germs get transmitted to you? A person who commutes each day in a packed subway car and then shares a cubicle with the mother of a three-year-old confronts different germs from a nurse working in the intensive care unit. As you let your mind walk through a typical day, you'll identify numerous places where germs might be transmitted.

➤ Susceptibility of the host: Are you just getting over a cold? Have you been working long hours, skipping meals,

Infections and Disease

In 1970, biochemist Linus Pauling touted vitamin C (ascorbic acid) in high doses as prevention for the common cold. At megadoses of 1 gram a day, Pauling believed the vitamin would decrease the number of colds a person would get in a lifetime.

Vitamin C is an essential nutrient needed by the body to make collagen. This compound strengthens blood vessel walls, connective tissue, and bone. Vitamin C is also an antioxidant that protects cell membranes.

The evidence on vitamin C's role in colds has been controversial and debated. Despite Pauling's strong belief in its benefits, he provided little scientific proof to back up his theory. Megadoses of any vitamin are not helpful to the body and can cause harm in some circumstances. Since the 1970s, the vitamin C-common cold connection has lost stature in medicine.

and missing sleep? Do you smoke? Do you exercise along a country road, in a crowded gym, or not at all? Without having much medical knowledge, you can probably make a pretty accurate assessment of your health, and, as a result, your susceptibility to infection.

➤ Exit from the host: This is critical for a pathogen's survival, but it affects you too. Give thought to your family. Are there infants in diapers? Pets? Consider your sex partner and the intimate contact involved. Do you work in a day care center or an emergency room? These questions all relate to pathogen exits from their hosts.

Taking Care of High-Risk Individuals

All links in the infection chain become more critical to manage when caring for someone at high risk for infection. These high-risk groups were described in Chapter 2.

A high-risk person is one who has a higher-than-normal susceptibility to infection. This may come about because of weakened immunity, underlying disease, age, or genetics. Other factors, such as gender, sometimes play a role. For whatever reason, the person in your care needs extra attention to fight infection. Some or all of the following steps might be appropriate:

➤ Provide dedicated bedding, towels, and bathroom articles (toothbrush, comb, razor, clippers, etc.)

➤ Treat wounds, cuts, and other broken skin with antiseptic while wearing disposable gloves; apply a bandage that covers the entire wound

➤ Clean and disinfect the person's bathroom sink, toilet bowl, floor, and shower weekly

➤ Clean and disinfect kitchen surfaces, handles, and floor weekly

➤ Use a water purification device for drinking water

➤ Use the sanitizer cycle in the dishwasher

➤ Do not serve raw milk, raw eggs, raw fish or shellfish, or rare meat

➤ Do not reuse a tasting spoon in a meal prepared for the high-risk person

➤ Avoid organic foods that cannot be peeled or cooked

➤ Provide gloves for gardening and spending time with pets

➤ Ensure that family members and close friends have up-to-date immunizations

➤ Follow doctor's recommendations for immunizations for the high-risk person

Infections and Disease

An extract of the echinacea herb has long been used to fight a variety of infections. It is a popular treatment for colds, and proponents recommend it be taken at the first signs of a cold to make the symptoms less severe.

Despite many studies on echinacea, doctors have yet to come to a consensus on its benefits. It may boost immunity, and like many herbs, its extract inhibits various microbes. No evidence exists that suggests echinacea is unsafe.

Risky Behavior and Infection

Some healthy individuals increase their chance of infection by adopting certain risky behaviors. Risky behavior ranges from sharing everyday items that probably carry your germs or the germs of others to more serious actions such as having unprotected sex. Vehicle transmission is an efficient way to exchange germs, and some bacteria and viruses can remain infectious on an inanimate surface for three or four days.

Following are some commonly shared items that can lead to infection:

➤ Water bottles

➤ Towels

➤ Lip balm

➤ Razors

➤ Toothbrushes

➤ Eating utensils

➤ Drinking glasses

➤ Clothes

➤ Hats

➤ Cosmetics

Other risky behavior involves activities that weaken immunity. Smoking, alcoholism, poor nutrition, and insufficient hours of sleep do this. After reading this book, you will probably be better at spotting risky behavior when you see it.

Microbe Basics

The term *nanobacteria* was coined in 1993 when a University of Texas geologist made a discovery in rocks retrieved from Italian hot springs. Using an electron microscope, he found tiny fossils of what looked like miniature bacteria. These fossils were 100 times smaller than normal bacteria. While most bacteria measure about 2 to 5 micrometers across, the nanobacteria fossils were only 10 to 200 nanometers in diameter.

A flurry of excitement rippled through scientific circles over the new bacteria. What role did these new bacteria play? Five years later the hubbub grew when two Finnish microbiologists found nanometer-sized bacteria in their lab. They felt the nanobacteria were related to the pathogens *Brucella* and *Bartonella*. This information caused consternation among microbiologists whose job it was to watch out for pathogens in medical patients. How could they be expected to find something so small?

In the years since these findings, few others have jumped on the nano bandwagon. Evidence is building to suggest the original nano-sized fossils did not represent bacteria. Other nanobacteria experiments have shown that large molecules can form aggregates that look like tiny bacteria but never become independent living things.

The worry over a new and barely detectable pathogen has subsided. Nanobacteria may exist; other, more impossible-to-believe discoveries have proven true. But for now, you need not stay up at night worrying about nano-pathogens.

At the Doctor's Office

The U.S. Food and Drug Administration (FDA) began protecting U.S. residents against ineffective or dangerous medicines and tainted foods with the passage in 1906 of the Pure Food and Drug Act. Since then, the Department of Health and Human Services enforces laws that ensure safe and effective drugs in addition to having other responsibilities regarding food safety.

The FDA oversees the testing of antibiotics and other treatments for infection in humans and animals. It offers resources on antibiotics, antibiotic resistance, and food-borne pathogens.

Do Alternative Treatments Work?

Some doctors feel alternative treatments put people at risk for various health problems. Alternative treatments are treatments that use substances that have not been tested or approved for medical use by the U.S. Food and Drug Administration (FDA). Treatments that fall into this category are homeopathy,

Chinese herbal medicines, Native American medicines, chiropractic treatments, and macrobiotic diets. More than two hundred alternative approaches to maintaining health are used in the United States.

A drug that has not been tested by the FDA may still be an effective treatment for a health condition. Many of the traditional medicines, or Eastern medicines, originated centuries before the FDA came into being. The evidence supporting some of these medicines as effective and safe may outweigh the data collected on newer western medicines.

Talk to a trusted doctor who listens to you. Discuss the pros and cons of alternative medicines and decide for yourself if they are worth a try. You must find a way of separating the myths from the facts. For some alternative products, you can be sure the manufacturer's desire to make money will lead to misleading claims.

Infections and Disease

Zinc is an essential nutrient needed by some of the body's enzymes. This mineral is also sold in over-the-counter (nonprescription) products for colds. Zinc-containing throat lozenges are the most common.

Zinc deficiency weakens immunity, as do many other nutrient deficiencies. During colds, zinc is thought to bind to rhinovirus and make it harder for the virus to attach to mucous membranes in the nose. Studies on zinc lozenges suggest it lessens the symptoms of colds, but scientific evidence has yet to prove that zinc helps cure the common cold.

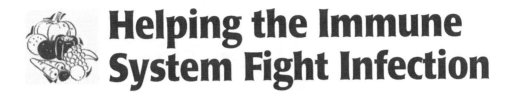

CHAPTER 18

Helping the Immune System Fight Infection

In This Chapter

➤ A review of the immune system

➤ Boosting immunity with good nutrition

➤ Boosting immunity with exercise and lower stress

➤ The medicines that help immunity

In this chapter you will learn ways to boost your body's immune system. Keeping strong and healthy and practicing good nutrition and hygiene are your best defenses against germs. This chapter covers the things everyone should do to help their body fight infection.

Three Ways to Fight Infection

The best way to fight infection is to stay healthy. I'm not trying to trick you with riddles. The immune system works behind the scenes every day fighting off potential infections. It can only do this at its optimum if you provide the fuel. The immune system needs nutrients to rebuild itself continually, but all other systems in the body also must be maintained at their peak. No one system or single organ should be allowed to falter and pull resources from other body systems.

Of course, this is not a perfect world. Even after doing your best, you might still catch a cold or get injured. Suddenly, the body must reassign resources to heal itself. Just like that, you're operating at suboptimal levels. Think what happens if a disease much more serious than a cold enters your body.

The best you can do every day is try to minimize risk to your body. This begins with good nutrition, exercise, reducing stress, and avoiding damaging activities like smoking and drinking excessive amounts of alcohol.

Fighting infection needs two additional steps, one preventive and one responsive. Keeping up to date on immunizations is a way to prevent many infections. By eliminating some infections by getting a vaccine, you become better prepared to fight the unexpected pathogens that come your way.

If a pathogen should manage to get past all your defenses and outwit the vaccine, you have a final weapon: a drug to kill the infectious agent. This means antibiotics, antiviral, antifungal and similar medicines.

This chapter focuses on the first way to prevent infections: nutrition, exercise, and stress reduction. If you keep your body at its best, then when you catch the inevitable germ, you'll fight it better.

At the Doctor's Office

Stress is a poorly understood condition in which an organism's normal systems go out of balance. Doctors call it disturbed equilibrium. One consequence of disturbed equilibrium is a weak immune response against infection. Infection itself plays a large role in putting a person into a stressed condition. Other known stressors are malnutrition, chronic disease, physical injury and pain, and psychological strain. All of these stressors increase susceptibility to infection.

Microbes can be stressed just as humans can, and this is the principle behind using antimicrobial products and food preservatives. Chemicals that stress microbes also weaken them so that the body has a better chance of stopping an infection.

Focusing on Your Body's Defenses

You cannot control the genetic component of your immunity, but you can control the health of every other part of your immune system.

The most basic parts of the body's defenses are cells and proteins. These make up skin, mucous membranes, white blood cells, antibodies, auxiliary proteins such as complement, and lymph.

Several organs support the defense components listed above. These are bone, the thymus, lymph nodes, and the spleen.

Bone

Bone marrow acts as the site for most of the cells that fight infection. Bone marrow supports the immune system in the following ways:

➤ Stem cells differentiate into red blood cells and platelets, which both have a part in blood clotting.

➤ Stem cells also turn into myeloblasts and monoblasts. Myeloblasts become white blood cells called granulocytes. You've already met the granulocytes. They are the eosinophils, basophils, and neutrophils. Monoblasts meanwhile develop into macrophages.

➤ Another type of stem cell creates cells that work in the lymphatic system: T lymphocytes and B lymphocytes. They also go by the names, T-cells and B-cells, respectively.

There's no need to feel confused. Just remember that you need healthy bone to make almost all of the blood cells that keep you free from infection.

Infection Vocabulary

The term *complement* refers to more than thirty different proteins that circulate in the bloodstream and participate in the body's response to infection. The complement system is activated when an antibody first binds with a foreign substance in the body. The proteins then help immunity in three ways: they strengthen the activity of antibodies, they enhance a variety of other immune reactions, and they help remove wastes produced in inflammation.

Thymus

The thymus gland is located above and slightly behind the heart. This is the main site where T-cells mature. T-cells can stay in the thymus, circulate in the blood, or go to the spleen and lymph nodes. T-cells are responsible for different complex reactions that control how immune cells react when an infectious agent invades the body.

Lymph Nodes and Spleen

Lymph is a fluid that moves through the body outside the bloodstream. Thousands of small kidney-shaped bulbs sit on the lymph vessels throughout the body. These are lymph nodes, which act to clean debris out of the lymph fluid. The debris is a mixture of destroyed microbial cells and used up immune cells.

The spleen is an organ in the abdomen. In a fetus, the spleen makes the baby's red and white blood cells. After birth, this organ behaves like a giant lymph node. It clears cell debris from blood and lymph fluid.

The liver, kidney, and brain also have specialized functions in immunity, and their health is vital to strong infection fighting. The circulatory system cannot be forgotten, either. Its vessels carry infection-fighting substances to the infection site. Thus anything that keeps the artery walls strong has a role in immunity.

At the Doctor's Office

Another word for the body's urge to maintain normal equilibrium is *homeostasis*. Literally, this means keeping a constant state. Your body makes continual discreet adjustments every minute to the external forces around it such as temperature, noise, and light. It does the same thing internally by monitoring blood levels of sugar, other nutrients, body temperature, heart rate, perspiration, etc. All of this monitoring and adjusting adds up to your personal homeostasis.

When you are free of infection, well nourished, and well rested, homeostasis is easy to maintain. But stresses put an added burden on the body to maintain homeostasis. In worst case scenarios, the body cannot maintain the balance and a disease such as cancer starts.

Fighting infection is a normal part of homeostasis. You should be able to imagine how infection that takes hold in the body disrupts homeostasis and can lead to more serious consequences.

Nutrition Basics

Good nutrition is required for cells of the immune system and all the supporting tissues so that they can rebuild, grow, strengthen, and carry out their jobs in the body.

The nutrients we need build cells, cells make tissue, and tissue comes together to make an organ. When we eat a meal, we are really giving the body the building blocks for making new membranes, proteins, enzymes, genetic material, and the milieu that fills cells.

It seems like extra work, but that's how metabolism does it. You eat proteins, carbohydrates, and other stuff so the body can break them down and remake them into proteins, carbohydrates, and other stuff. Nutrients also provide another need: energy. Part of our intake goes to powering the cell systems in every organ.

Let's learn the basics of the nutrients from which the immune system and all other systems are built.

Carbohydrates, Proteins, and Fats

These three types of nutrients make up most of your diet. They all contain mainly carbon, oxygen, and hydrogen. Many types also have nitrogen, sulfur, and phosphorus. Meet the carbohydrates, proteins, and fats in more detail:

➤ Carbohydrates: Includes sugars, starches, and glycogen. These compounds are used for energy to power all body systems. Carbohydrates provide structure to cells and tissue, store ready-to-use energy, and are part of glycoproteins. Glycoproteins attach to the outside of the body's cells and help the cell communicate with its surroundings. This role is especially important in the immune system, where white blood cells must recognize foreign matter.

➤ Protein: Made of strings of amino acids, proteins make up the support structure of cells, act as enzymes, and build muscles. Antibodies and many of the substances that help regulate the immune response are proteins. These substances include complement, cytokines, and interleukin.

➤ Certain tasks carried out in the immune system could not happen without protein. The body needs twenty different amino acids, called the essential amino acids, to build the proteins it needs. By eating protein from a variety of sources (meat, nuts, eggs, milk, etc.), you get the essential amino acids in an amount sufficient to make your own protein.

➤ Fats: The main energy storage form in the body, fats are also a key component in membranes. This group includes the essential oils, omega-3 fatty acids, and sterol. The body uses sterol to make vitamin D, which helps maintain membrane health and skin health.

Vitamins

Vitamins are auxiliary nutrients; they help with the metabolism of carbohydrates, proteins, and fats. Biologists divide them into two groups: fat-soluble and water-soluble. Fat-soluble vitamins are vitamins A, D, E, and K. The water-soluble members are the B vitamins and vitamin C.

Each vitamin has a unique set of functions in the body, which can be quite extensive. In general, vitamins serve the following major functions to keep cells running:

> ➤ Maintain membranes
>
> ➤ Help enzymes work
>
> ➤ Function in body pigments for energy generation and sight
>
> ➤ Help maintain nerve function
>
> ➤ Aid in nutrient absorption
>
> ➤ Serve as precursors to other compounds made by the body
>
> ➤ Act in blood clotting

Minerals

A mineral is an inorganic element, such as iron, copper, and magnesium. Minerals are the only nutrients the body uses that are not of animal or plant origin.

Minerals are also auxiliary nutrients. Sometimes minerals help vitamins do their job. For example, vitamin B12 does not work unless it has a cobalt atom at its center. In other instances, a mineral enables an enzyme to carry out its tasks in the body. When minerals play an auxiliary role in enzyme reactions, they are called cofactors.

Calcium and Phosphorus

Calcium and phosphorus are important in maintaining the body's health. Calcium builds new bone, helps the mammary gland make milk, works with enzymes, helps with blood clotting, and plays an essential role in nerve and muscle function. Calcium is so important to the body that it is required in amounts higher than other minerals.

Phosphorus is a key player in energy use and in the uptake of other nutrients by the digestive tract. DNA cannot be made without phosphorus.

Nutrition for Adults and Children

Nutrient requirements are the minimum amount of each nutrient needed by the body for good health. These requirements are based on an average person, so you may need a little more or a little less, depending on your body type.

Too much of a good thing does not lead to better nutrition. An excess of carbohydrates, proteins, and fats leads to weight gain. Vitamin and mineral excesses cause a variety of disorders that can be even more dangerous to your health than deficiencies.

As a rule of thumb, excess intake of fat-soluble vitamins is more dangerous than excess intake of water-soluble vitamins. Fat-soluble vitamins go to the body's fat stores and accumulate there. Taking extra vitamin A for example accumulates in fatty tissue until it reaches toxic levels. Excess water-soluble vitamins are eliminated in the kidneys and are excreted in urine.

Maintaining Healthy Skin

Since the skin is the first line of defense, it makes sense to start your nutrition for fighting infections here.

Nutrient deficiencies show up as dry, cracked skin, a situation that can be disastrous for keeping out opportunistic pathogens. Feeding the skin does not differ from keeping any other part of the body nourished, but some nutrients seem to have special benefits to skin and include the following:

➤ Omega-3 and essential fatty acids: Supplied in the fat portion of your diet, these substances help maintain the skin's moisture content and production of normal secretions, such as sebum. The secretions aid in repelling many unwanted microbes that land on the skin.

➤ Antioxidants such as selenium and vitamins A, C, and E: These nutrients protect living skin layers and underlying connective tissue from destruction by normal by-products of metabolism.

➤ Zinc: This mineral helps several enzyme systems work properly. It also participates in oil production in skin glands and aids hormone function. Hormones affect the health of skin in various ways.

Keeping Blood Healthy

The blood carries oxygen to your cells, totes away wastes, and transports the immune system players that fight infection. Who wouldn't want to have the healthiest blood possible?

Following are the main nutrients that have a direct effect on blood health:

➤ Iron: Functions as the oxygen carrier in hemoglobin

➤ Protein: Makes other essential proteins such as antibodies, cytokines, interleukins, etc.; and hemoglobin, a protein in red blood cells that carries oxygen everywhere blood goes in your body

➤ Vitamin B12 and cobalt: Makes hemoglobin; B12 cannot do its job without the mineral cobalt (Consult a nutritionist to see if you're getting enough B12. There should be no need to take a cobalt supplement; all diets provide plenty of this nutrient.)

➤ Vitamin K: Helps with the formation of blood clots to wall off infections from the rest of the body; vitamin K is one of several required blood-clotting factors

Helping the Lymphatic System

The lymphatic system needs the same balanced nutrient supply as the rest of your body. Since lymph fluid and the system's vessels contain proteins, this nutrient should be at the top of your list. Otherwise, the lymphatic system works best with a well-rounded supply of carbohydrates, proteins, and fats, plus the essential vitamins and minerals.

All body systems require micronutrients, so-called because the body uses them in very small amounts. Without these nutrients, certain enzymes do not function. Without enzymes, your normal metabolism slows down. Somewhere in this cascade of events, immunity begins to falter.

Do not plan on supplementing your diet with pills full of micronutrients without first consulting a nutrition expert. This kind of supplementation has a better chance of harming you than helping. A balanced diet of meats and fish, carbohydrates and grains, and fruits and vegetables deliver all the micronutrients you need. In case you're wondering, these are the micronutrients:

➤ Iron

➤ Zinc

➤ Selenium

➤ Iodine (as iodide)

➤ Copper

➤ Manganese

➤ Molybdenum

➤ Fluorine (as fluoride)

➤ Chromium

These are additional micronutrients that the body may need, but researchers have not yet confirmed:

➤ Boron

➤ Nickel

➤ Vanadium

➤ Arsenic

➤ Silicon

Micronutrients are minerals, so nutritionists sometimes refer to them as trace minerals or trace nutrients.

No single nutrient acts like a magic bullet for boosting your immunity. Don't listen to any dietary claims that suggest a nutrient boosts immunity beyond what a well-planned and complete diet can do.

Exercise

You will probably never have enough time or money to read all the books on how to enhance immunity through diet, exercise, and reducing stress. Just trying to read them all might increase your stress levels!

The exercise-immunity connection is a relatively recent area of study. Medical researchers and proponents of alternative medicines and diets can agree on this one thing: exercise at the proper levels can only benefit your health and stress levels and therefore strengthen your immunity.

Exercise increases your heart rate and gets blood moving through your body. This automatically increases the circulation of immune system cells. Greater circulation of these cells increases the chances that they will find and destroy foreign invaders faster.

Scientific studies have also uncovered evidence that exercise speeds antibody production and quickens the response of certain T-cells to infection. To get this benefit, exercise for twenty to thirty minutes five days a week. The exercises you choose should increase your heart rate. Consult a doctor for a regimen best suited to you.

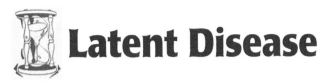

CHAPTER 19

Latent Disease

In This Chapter

➤ Latent diseases compared with slow and persistent infections

➤ The main latent diseases we get

➤ An introduction to latent TB infection

In this chapter you will see one of the ways in which pathogens evade the immune system. Despite the efficiency of the human immune system, pathogens wouldn't be where there are today without effective countermeasures. One way to evade the immune system is to find a hiding place in the body and sit there silently until the coast is clear. This is the basic premise behind latency.

Latency is a state of being concealed or inactive. A latent disease is one in which a pathogen goes inactive or dormant shortly after infecting the body and stays that way for a long time. Latent periods can last for several years to several decades.

Latent infections frustrate patients and doctors alike. You may think you have done everything right to avoid infection, but many years later you find out that the pathogen had been inside you all along. It sounds like good science fiction but is actually another example of how well pathogens have adapted to the hosts they infect.

Pathogens that Cause Latent Infections

Latent diseases are usually caused by viruses. Viruses are exquisitely suited for latency because they do not grow. Rather, viruses exist inside other living cells. Since the modus operandi of a virus is to hide inside a host cell, why not hide a while longer until the immune cells go away, and then create havoc? This approach works well for several viruses that cause common infections in our society.

An unusual bacterium that causes latent infection is called the latent TB organism. Latent TB can be distinguished from the regular form of the disease, called active TB, because it doesn't cause symptoms. Both diseases are caused by *Mycobacterium tuberculosis*. Only about 10 percent of people infected with latent TB will develop the normal symptoms of TB. The chance of developing symptoms rise in people with weakened immune systems, especially AIDS patients, organ transplant recipients, and cancer patients.

The discussion of latent diseases and similar slow-developing diseases begins with viruses.

Slow and Persistent Viruses

Three different groups of viruses behave differently in the human body, but all have in common a very slow course of infection. Slow viruses and persistent viruses are sometimes confused with latent viruses, but each has its distinctions.

Infections and Disease

Persistent viral infections are rare and tend to affect the nervous system. The main examples of these infections in humans are: subacute sclerosing panencephalitis (SSPE) from measles infection, which causes mental deterioration; progressive encephalitis from rubella virus infection, which causes rapid mental deterioration; and progressive multifocal leukoencephalopathy from papovavirus infection, which causes brain degeneration.

Persistent secondary infections are also seen in AIDS. The dementia associated with AIDS comes from persistent infections from various viruses, including herpes, echovirus, and the HIV itself.

Slow viruses create diseases in which the symptoms take a long time to develop. The slow virus may not necessarily go dormant in the body during this time.

Measles is the best-known example of a disease caused by a slow virus. The rubeola virus enters the body via the respiratory tract and causes symptoms of measles soon afterward: fever, sneezing, nasal congestion, harsh cough, general malaise, and papules that erupt on the skin over the entire body. The disease begins to resolve after about ten days, but five to twelve years later, the person can develop a slow degenerative brain disease from the same virus, which remained in the body. This disease is subacute sclerosing panencephalitis (SSPE). This disease may cause permanent nerve damage and death.

Persistent viruses cause diseases in which the symptoms appear soon after infection, but remain for many years. These diseases also fall into the general category of chronic disease, which is a category of diseases that last a long time in the body. (The opposite is an acute infection in which symptoms appear quickly and leave quickly.) Persistent infections endure because the immune system cannot eliminate the virus from the body however hard it tries.

Infectious mononucleosis is a persistent disease caused by the Epstein-Barr virus. In this disease, a sufferer experiences sore throat, fever, and swollen lymph nodes after a period of one to seven weeks, and then the virus enters a longer-lasting period by hiding in immune system cells. For reasons not fully understood, the virus becomes active again and causes an acute hepatitis. Some virologists refer to Epstein-Barr's nonpathogenic period as a dormant period. This highlights the confusion that can arise when trying to distinguish slow, persistent, and latent viruses.

The following sections discuss the most common viruses known to enter long periods of latency before symptoms of disease appear.

Microbe Basics

Incubation period lasts from the moment a pathogen infects your body to the moment the first symptoms of infection appear. Incubation periods are usually characteristic of a pathogen and can last hours, days, or weeks.

Incubation is a busy time for a pathogen, although you are unaware of its presence. During the incubation period, the pathogen overcomes the body's initial defenses and often moves through the body in search of its preferred target tissue. Then, the pathogen begins multiplying to numbers large enough to overcome any additional waves of assault from the immune system. The incubation period represents a critical time in infection when the scales can tip either in the pathogen's favor or in yours.

Chickenpox and Shingles

The disease chickenpox also goes by the name varicella and is caused by the varicella-zoster virus. It usually infects children under age fifteen, but it is not confined to the young.

Varicella uses droplet transmission and enters through the respiratory tract. People can also get the infection by touching an open pustule of an infected child's rash. Chickenpox's incubation period is two to three weeks. The symptoms include fever, malaise, loss of appetite, and a characteristic itchy rash. The rash covers the face, trunk, scalp, thighs, and upper arms.

People who recover from chickenpox have immunity for life. The virus, however, stays in the body inside nerve cells. The varicella-zoster strips down during this period to a single piece of viral DNA, which it mixes with the host nerve cell's DNA.

During this latent period, no one can detect that you have the virus. Certain stresses years later may activate the viral DNA and new viruses may begin to form. Being immunocompromised is one of the known reasons that varicella-zoster reappears in the body. AIDS patients, organ transplant recipients, cancer patients, and people with neurological disorders all have a higher risk of varicella-zoster awakening from dormancy.

The reactivated form of chickenpox is the disease called shingles. (To keep you in a prolonged state of confusion, the virus becomes known as herpes zoster at this point!) Shingles appears most often in people over fifty years old. This painful ailment is characterized by a recurring rash.

Chickenpox is highly contagious and hard to avoid. The best way to avoid chickenpox is to get it and recover from it when young! A generation ago, parents kept all children in their family together as soon as one showed symptoms of chickenpox. This ensured that their children would all be free from chickenpox for life.

Today, many parents are more inclined to opt for vaccination against chickenpox. The chickenpox vaccine is given in two doses to children who have never been infected. The first dose is at twelve to fifteen months of age, and the booster shot is given at four to six years of age. Similar two-dose vaccines about six weeks apart can also be given to anyone thirteen years or older.

A shingles vaccine has become increasing popular for Baby Boomers who got through chickenpox in their youth. It is not 100 percent effective in preventing shingles, but lessens the effects of the disease in most people who get the vaccine.

Herpes

Herpes is a complex conglomeration of infections caused by different forms of the herpes virus. Herpes simplex virus types 1 and 2 (HSV-1 and HSV-2) attack mucous membranes on the genitals and other places on the body. After getting through this barrier, the virus finds nerve cells and migrates along the nerve fibers in the direction of sensory ganglia. Sensory ganglia are tangles of nerves that receive information from your senses (sight, hearing, touch, etc.) and route the information to the brain. Think of intricate highway interchanges outside big cities.

The herpes virus settles into the ganglia for its latent period until reactivated by stress, fever, sex, or exposure to sunlight. (The ultraviolet light in sunlight is responsible for this activation.) Then, the virus retraces its trail to the initial infection site, causing blisters (fever blisters). During the period in which the blisters are apparent, the herpes patient is highly contagious.

As you expect by now, herpes infection is worse in immunocompromised people. In these cases, it travels deeper into the nervous system to the brain and the meninges. Headaches, fevers, seizures, and an altered mental state ensue. These events may be partly responsible for symptoms seen in AIDS patients. The antiviral drug acyclovir helps treat herpes infections.

At the Doctor's Office

Two types of measles exist. Measles is the infection caused by the rubeola virus, whereas the German measles is caused by the rubella virus. German measles creates a red rash on the skin that lasts no more than three days, when the virus then disappears from the body. German measles can be serious if it occurs in pregnant women, but otherwise this disease has a low incidence in the United States and is not a public health concern.

HIV

HIV has a long latency period that culminates with the emergence in the body of the disease AIDS. HIV-1 is the most common type of the virus in the United States and the type that started the AIDS epidemic here in the 1980s. AIDS was unknown in the United States before 1982 but is now a worldwide epidemic. The majority of people with AIDS are between the ages of fifteen and forty-five, poor, and heterosexual. The disease is devastating communities in sub-Saharan Africa and Asia.

HIV-1 and the second type, HIV-2, infect through mucous membranes during sexual contact and also enter the bloodstream with the use of contaminated needles. HIV-2 predominates in Africa.

HIV's latency occurs both in immune system T-cells and in nerve cells. In these places, the virus cannot be reached by drug treatments.

Like other latent viruses, HIV disassembles itself inside the host cell and puts its DNA into the host cell's DNA. The trigger for HIV emergence from latency is not fully known.

No cure for AIDS exists at this time. New treatments for interfering with HIV's multiplication in the body have been marginally successful. This infection is avoided best by reducing the number of your sexual partners and using a condom during sex.

Hepatitis B

Hepatitis B virus (HBV) causes a latent form of hepatitis, which is inflammation of the liver. Like herpes and HIV, HBV is a sexually transmitted infection but can be transmitted in other ways. People get this virus by being exposed to contaminated blood or body fluids. Blood transfusions, contaminated medical equipment, nonsterile needles, and body secretions (sweat, saliva, semen, etc.) have transmitted HBV.

HBV's latent period is a relatively short two to six months, but evidence is mounting that this virus can be dormant for much longer periods. It hides in liver cells, where the symptoms also occur at the time of the disease.

HBV has limited drug therapy, mainly drugs that are still in clinical testing. An HBV vaccine is effective and taken mainly by healthcare workers.

Latent TB

Let's take a closer look at a bacterium unusual because it causes a latent disease.

People with the latent form of *M. tuberculosis* give positive results when they take the tuberculin skin test for the presence of the pathogen. However, they seldom develop symptoms and do not transmit TB to others. Infected people have no signs of lesions in the lungs in X-rays, even though such lesions are a hallmark of this disease in regular TB patients.

At the Doctor's Office

The Mantoux tuberculin skin test serves as a standard way for your doctor to tell if you have ever been exposed to the TB pathogen. In this simple test, a nurse injects a small amount of protein that had been purified from *Mycobacterium* under skin in your forearm. Within forty-eight to seventy-two hours, a person's immune system will form a hardening around the injection site that indicates previous infection with TB.

This test does not tell the doctor whether the TB infection is happening now or occurred some time ago. People with a positive result in the Mantoux test receive drug treatment.

TB is a serious disease, and because of its risks, people diagnosed with latent TB receive the same treatment as those with regular or active TB. The drug regimen consists of four drugs at varying doses alternating between daily and twice weekly. The treatment is similar to that of active TB and has the following four phases:

> ➤ Take isoniazid for nine months

> ➤ Take a lowered dose of isoniazid for an additional six months

> ➤ Take rifampin for four months

> ➤ Take rifampicin and pyrazinamide (optional)

Immunocompromised people, health care workers, and people living in regions of the world where TB is prevalent are at higher risk for being infected by both kinds of TB. TB is transmitted only by droplet contact transmission, so you need not worry about getting infected from inanimate objects or even from touching another person who has TB.

CHAPTER 20

Antibodies and Immunity

In This Chapter

➤ Overview of the role of antibodies in adaptive immunity

➤ An introduction to antigens and their effect on the body

➤ Types of antibodies and how they work

➤ Things you can do to boost your antibodies

In this chapter we explore the part of the immune system unique to each one of us. Antibodies are proteins made by the body to fight specific infectious agents. These proteins are so focused on the pathogen they were made to find, that they pass right by other microbes in the body. Since each one of us is exposed to a unique array of microbes in a lifetime, no two people will have the same antibody makeup.

Antibodies are the stars of the immune system. They belong to the arm of immunity called adaptive immunity. The word *adaptive* may give you an idea of how this part of immunity works. Imagine a soccer game in which the goalkeeper isn't allowed to move his feet. He deflects any shots within reach, but a strong opponent can stretch him to his limits and score almost at will. Picture now a goalie who is allowed to move her feet when defending the goal. She dives, she stretches, and sometimes she jumps to catch the shot; other times she kicks the ball away. The stationary goalie is a bit like your innate defenses; stout but unchangeable. The mobile goalie is like your adaptive defenses, which responds to whatever life throws at it. And the cornerstone to that adaptability is the antibody.

Overview of Adaptive Immunity

The more you know about immunity, the more I hope you'll appreciate the elegance of this defense against infection. The entire immune system contains parts that cooperate, complement, and back up each other. If one member falters, a second or even a third member of the immune system steps up to confront the infectious agent.

Adaptive immunity contains cell- and antibody-mediated responses to infection. The antibody part of your immune system is called humoral immunity. It was named for the body's humors, which centuries ago were thought to confer health on a person through a mysterious mix of biology and spirituality.

Biologists credit antibodies with giving us acquired immunity because humans must develop or acquire them over time. Everyone acquires their antibodies in four ways:

➤ Your mother passes some to you through the placenta while you are a fetus.

➤ Your mother gives you more in colostrum, the first breast milk you drink when nursing.

➤ You develop antibodies on your own as you become exposed to antigens.

➤ You develop antibodies after receiving vaccinations for common childhood diseases or other vaccines later in life.

Antibodies cannot form unless a foreign substance appears in the body. This foreign thing could be a microbe or other small biological entity, and it is called an antigen. Anything that was not made by your body but is now circulating in your bloodstream or lodged in your tissues is an antigen.

Antigens are microscopic and don't include foreign matter such as prosthetic devices, but even these devices can elicit a defense response from the immune system.

Infection Vocabulary

Colostrum is breast fluid that is secreted from the second trimester onward, but it is most evident in the first two to three days after giving birth. Colostrum appears before regular lactation begins. This fluid supplies the infant with a concentrated dose of immunoglobulins to boost the newborn's immune system while also providing other proteins and calories. The immunoglobulins from colostrum give the baby immunity for only a few weeks, so they serve as merely short-term protection.

It is impossible to think about antibodies without also learning something about antigens. Let's begin with antigens since they start the whole antibody-producing process in motion when they come in contact with your body.

Antigens

The purpose of the immune system is to differentiate the matter in your body between self and nonself. Before you are born, your body inventories all of its different types of cells. Your immune system, though immature, remembers the details of these various tissue types and labels them Self.

From the perspective of the immune system, the moment you're born you begin a journey through life that is under constant assault by all sorts of unwanted junk. Any junk that makes close contact with the skin or gets inside the body will be identified as nonself. These nonself materials are what immunologists call antigens. Here are some typical antigens:

Infection Vocabulary

You might see in some articles on antibodies and antigens the symbols Ab and An. These are simply shorthand for any antibody and antigen, respectively.

> ➤ Proteins

> ➤ Polysaccharides

> ➤ Glycolipids (lipid molecules with a sugar attached)

> ➤ Egg whites

> ➤ Blood cells from other people or species

> ➤ Serum proteins from other people or species

> ➤ Substances on the surface of transplanted tissue or organs

> ➤ Pollens

> ➤ Microbes

Every antigen has some unique substances on its surface that makes it identifiable in a chemical sense. These identifying marks are called epitopes.

When any antigen is in your body, the immune system has a process for detecting it. Messages go out to alert the body of the foreigner's presence. Lymphocytes called B-cells receive the message and start making antibodies. The antibodies they make have sections that are constructed to connect with the antigen's epitopes similar to the way a lock and key fit together. Biologists in fact refer to the binding of antibody to antigen as a lock-and-key complex. Whether the antigen is a short strand of protein or a large hunk of pollen, an antibody clutches it in a tight hold until other members of the immune system can arrive and destroy the foreigner.

Remember, antigens can cause the immune system to react to them even if they do not get inside the body. Many different types of rashes are really reactions to an antigen on the skin. Rashes that are caused by immune events rather than other types of irritation are often accompanied by fever, joint pains, and malaise (a general sense of feeling lousy).

Microbe Basics

Microbiologists have figured out a way to identify pathogens in a sick person by studying the microbes' antigens. After taking a blood, sputum, or other type of sample from the person's body, the microbiologist mixes the sample with known antibodies that recognize specific pathogens. These antibodies can be purchased from laboratory supply companies.

After mixing the two together, a positive reaction between the antigen in the sample and pathogen A antibody tells the microbiologist that pathogen A caused the infection. A negative reaction between the antigen and antibodies for pathogens B, C, D, and so on means that those microbes could not have caused the infection.

The unique epitopes on pathogen A give it its serotype. A serotype is like your fingerprint. Serotyping allows microbiologists to diagnose disease and even trace the cause of food-borne infection.

Superantigens

Superantigens are foreign proteins that elicit an extra-big response by the immune system. The response is so drastic that the body harms itself in its efforts to destroy the superantigen.

Superantigens stimulate lymphocytes called T-cells to proliferate in the body. The T-cells in turn release an enormous amount of cytokines. Cytokines are important in a normally stimulated immune response, but at abnormally high levels in the bloodstream they cause uncomfortable reactions by the body. These reactions are usually fever, nausea, vomiting, and diarrhea.

Infection Vocabulary

Helper T-cells are lymphocytes that play equally important roles in the immune system's cellular response to infection and its antibody response to invaders. They are called T-cells because they originate in the thymus. The thymus is a glandlike structure at the base of the neck.

Helper T-cells make contact with an antigen even before B-cells detect the antigen. The T-cells then secrete cytokines to stimulate B-cells to produce antibodies. T-cells are multitaskers when it comes to immunity—they also stimulate the release of macrophages and the production of eosinophils. Four types of T-cells operate in different parts of the body. All types primarily target bacteria and viruses that infect the body.

In the most serious cases of cytokine release as a response to a superantigen, the body can go into shock and possibly die. Some of the illnesses caused by superantigens are toxic shock syndrome caused by *Staph aureus*, scarlet fever and rheumatic fever caused by *Streptococcus*, and certain *Staph*-caused food poisonings.

Because of the toxic effect of superantigens, these proteins have also been called type I toxins. Fortunately, your chances of being exposed to superantigens are much lower than being exposed to regular antigens.

Antibodies

Considering the diversity of things that act as antigens in the body, your chances of getting an antigen inside you sometime soon are very high. It's time to examine the other half of the lock-and-key connection, the antibody.

Antibodies are proteins, specifically immunoglobulin proteins. A globulin is a protein of blood serum. (Serum is the fluid portion of blood minus the red blood cells.) Globulins account for almost 40 percent of

Infection Vocabulary

What does the body do about all those millions of microbes on the skin, in the mouth, and in the intestines? Shouldn't those microbes prompt a dramatic immune response?

Our immune systems give our normal flora a free pass due to a feature called immune tolerance. Various complex systems feed information to the immune system to tell it that our normal flora is our friend. This immune tolerance begins when a person is still an embryo but becomes fully developed in following years.

all proteins in blood. The globulins devoted to a life chasing antigens throughout the body are immunoglobulins.

An immunoglobulin has a shape like the letter Y. The stem of the Y doesn't do much in immunity, but the two arms of the Y play a critical role. The end of each arm serves as a site for binding to an antigen, so one antibody has the capacity to bind two antigens.

How Antibodies Defend Us

Antibodies get rid of antigens in more than one way. Some antibodies can destroy the antigen with little help from the rest of the immune system. They can degrade toxins and even kill parasitic worms. Most others, however, hold onto the antigen and simultaneously send out a simple message: Help! Phagocytes hear the cry and circulate through the bloodstream until they find the antibody-antigen complex. When these cells arrive at the scene, they destroy the entire complex.

But how does an antibody manage to come up with a perfect lock-and-key coupling with an antigen it has never seen before? In truth, antibodies are a lot less effective in protecting you against new germs. Other parts of the immune system take the lead in this task. Antibodies give the body a type of memory for future infections by a pathogen that has infected you in the past. Indeed, the cells that produce antibodies are called memory B-cells.

Infection Vocabulary

B-cells are lymphocytes that mature in bone marrow, then migrate to the lymphatic system to work against infection. All B-cells develop specifically to produce an antibody to a unique antigen. B-cells serve the body best by congregating in the spleen and lymph nodes. Because a large volume of blood passes through these organs, B-cells can sit and watch the flow go by them. When they spot an antigen to which they make antibodies, the B-cells begin to multiply far beyond their normal numbers. During this proliferation, some B-cells become specialized memory B-cells. The memory B-cells take responsibility for making antibodies again in the future should the same antigen reappear.

The first time your body gets a particular antigen, it musters a primary antibody response. Antibodies don't show up until several days after the infection has started, and their ability to control the antigen can be fairly weak. The second time that the same antigen appears, the so-called secondary antibody response arises much faster and stronger. This is because memory B-cells gathered information about the antigen the first time around. They put together a blueprint for making antibodies specific to that antigen should it ever infect again. When that second infection occurs, your body is much better equipped to fight the infection. (Some T-cells also play the part of memory T-cells, but they do not make antibodies.)

Five classes of antibodies work in the body in slightly different ways. Each of these types also has certain antigens it prefers to attack. Let's see what they do.

Immunoglobulin G (IgG)

IgG antibodies account for 80 percent of all the antibodies in serum. Anything that is so predominant must be important.

IgG antibodies work in the bloodstream and squeeze through blood vessel walls to chase antigens in tissue. You receive these antibodies early; they cross the placental wall to the fetus during gestation.

These antibodies attach to bacteria and viruses and signal phagocytes to show up. They can also neutralize toxins by themselves and trigger the complement system. Complement proteins regulate the fine points of phagocytosis and the destruction of bacteria. IgG antibodies also stay in the blood longer than any other type of antibody. After twenty-three days following the initial infection, about half of IgG antibodies are still around.

Infection Vocabulary

You may read about a special type of cytokines called interleukins. Interleukins are proteins that help various white blood cells communicate with other cells. This communication allows the immune system to better coordinate its attack against infection.

Interleukins enable the body to launch a stronger defense against microbes and other foreign matter by regulating inflammation. These proteins also talk to muscle, liver, adrenal, and bone cells to regulate their activity during infection.

Immunoglobulin M (IgM)

IgM antibodies make up 5 to 10 percent of all antibodies. Think of the M in IgM as standing for "mega." IgM antibodies are composed of five regular Y-shaped antibodies connected at their stems with all the arms pointing outward in a circle. This structure enables IgM to bind with up to ten antigens.

IgM antibodies are big. They lumber through the bloodstream but cannot cross into tissue like IgG can. For their size, however, they are light on their feet. IgM is usually the first antibody to show up when an antigen appears.

Infection Vocabulary

Biologists learned many years ago that the very specific nature of antibodies could be put to good use. Antibodies can find a miniscule amount of antigen within a heterogeneous mixture of other substances. To take advantage of this ability, biologists produce monoclonal antibodies in special laboratories.

A monoclonal antibody is an artificial antibody made by B-cells that have been spliced together with cancer cells. The cancer cells contribute their special talent: enormously fast growth. (Monoclonal antibodies do not cause cancer.) The B-cells produce a specific antibody to a known antigen.

Monoclonal antibodies (MAb) have been used as treatments for rheumatoid arthritis, Crohn's disease, and non-Hodgkin's lymphoma. Several new monoclonal antibodies are being investigated for additional cancers.

IgM antibodies are the reason two different blood types can be incompatible in the body. When IgM sees red blood cells that don't match the ones in the body, it makes big clumps of the cells. This can be life-threatening if a person is transfused with the wrong blood type. In infection fighting, IgM antibodies behave like IgG antibodies by holding onto an antigen and helping phagocytes destroy it.

Because IgM is a first responder to infection, it serves as a good aid in diagnosis of the cause of the infection. But this diagnosis has to be done quickly; about five days after the infection starts, only about half of IgM remains.

Immunoglobulin A (IgA)

IgA antibodies also make up about 10 percent of all antibodies present at a given time in the blood. IgA is made of two Y-shaped antibodies attached by their stems so that this antibody can bind to four antigens.

IgA stays almost exclusively on mucous membranes and in mucus, saliva, tears, and breast milk. IgA protects you at the front lines of the body at the mucous membranes. It prevents bacteria and viruses from attaching there. This antibody is also abundant in colostrum and probably helps protect infants from diarrhea as bacteria from the outside world start entering the digestive tract.

The IgA in tears, saliva, and milk may have special duties not found in the IgA of mucous membranes. For this reason, it is called secretory IgA.

Like IgM, IgA does not stay active for long; most of it is gone about a week after being released into blood.

Immunoglobulin D (IgD)

IgD antibodies make up only 0.2 percent of antibodies. These antibodies stay mainly on the B-cells' surface. There, they help the B-cell recognize various antigens. Once a B-cell recognizes an antigen, it begins making the specific antibody to the antigen by fiddling with the composition at the ends of the Y.

Infection Vocabulary

The risk of autoimmune disease increases when the body loses its immune tolerance. Autoimmune disease is an illness in which the body's immune system attacks cells or tissues in its own body. Specifically, self-attacking antibodies, called autoantibodies, cause the trouble.

About eighty autoimmune diseases are now known; some of these have received more research than others. But the causes of autoimmune disease remain a puzzle. While scientists continue to search for the triggers to autoimmune disease, immunologists have determined some of the events that happen in an autoimmune disease. For instance, foreign antigens may be similar in structure to certain body cells. This fools the body into releasing substances that attack both. In other instances, part of a cell in your body combines with an antigen. The immune system cannot figure out whether this new hybrid is self or nonself. Finally, some T-cells contain an error that makes them start attacking the body's self tissues.

Many autoimmune diseases appear in periodic flare-ups of symptoms, then the symptoms go away for a while. Some of the most common autoimmune diseases prevalent in women (but can affect men) are multiple sclerosis, Graves' disease, type 1 diabetes, celiac disease, inflammatory bowel disease, and rheumatoid arthritis.

Immunoglobulin E (IgE)

IgE antibodies exist in the lowest percent of all antibodies, about 0.002 percent. IgE attaches its stem to basophils and other immune cells and participates in a special allergic reaction called the anaphylactic response.

Anaphylaxsis is an extreme allergic reaction called hypersensitivity. It is caused by a sudden release of a large amount of immune substances in response to particular antigens. This usually happens after a person has previously been exposed to the offending antigen. The antigen in this case is called an allergen. The most common causes of an anaphylactic reaction are certain drugs, food, pollen, and insect stings.

Infections and Disease

Rheumatic fever is an autoimmune disease that can develop after a throat infection by *Streptococcus* group A (strep throat) has persisted untreated. The disease is an overreaction by the immune system to superantigen proteins on the bacterial cell. Cytokines pour into the bloodstream in response. This sudden influx of cytokine leads to suppression of some immune reactions and possible toxicity. Two major outcomes of the disease are heart valve inflammations and arthritis.

How to Boost Your Antibodies

The immune system can get worn out when too many infections challenge it. Frequent barrages of antigens leave little time for the body to replenish white blood cells, lymphocytes, and antibodies.

The best way to support your antibody machinery is the same as supporting all other body systems: good nutrition, adequate rest, and reduced stress. Since antibodies are proteins, the body cannot make them in sufficient quantities if your diet lacks a balanced blend of essential amino acids. Protein synthesis also needs vitamins and minerals that enable protein-making enzymes to work. Chicken soup? Not a bad place to start.

CHAPTER 21

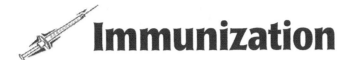 **Immunization**

In This Chapter

➤ An overview of immunization and vaccination

➤ How we receive natural immunization

➤ Different types of vaccines and how they are made

➤ Basic information on today's most-used vaccines

➤ Herd immunity, vaccine safety, and side effects

➤ The consequences of not immunizing yourself or your family

In this chapter you will learn about immunization. Immunization is the most controversial topic in infection fighting. Two divergent schools of thought exist with plenty of confused and worried people stuck in the middle.

On one hand, medical professionals have decades of evidence showing that immunization helps lower the incidence of many diseases that a century ago claimed thousands of lives. On the other hand, opponents of immunization programs worry over the safety of drugs made from the very pathogens that cause illness and death. Opponents cite also their concern over the side effects of injecting these substances into a healthy body.

With a background in antibodies from the preceding chapter, you will now learn how vaccines help your body make antibodies. By learning about the types of vaccines and how they are made, you can feel confident you know what is happening inside your body when you receive a vaccine.

Immunization and Vaccination

Immunization is the act of getting antibodies. Immunization behaves like a safety net for your body's lines of defense. In order to get the immunity against infection provided by immunization, you need a little help from others.

You can be naturally immunized by your mother before birth or after birth when you nurse. You may also be artificially immunized through vaccination. Vaccination is the injection of a substance into your body that either gives you antibodies outright or prompts you to make antibodies.

Since we tend to equate immunization with getting a shot, the terms *immunization* and *vaccination* have become used almost interchangeably.

Infections in History

No scientist contributed more to microbiology than Frenchman Louis Pasteur (1822–1895). Pasteur had an interest in vaccines and was the first microbiologist to experiment with attenuation. By injecting pathogens into animals, recovering the microbe, and repeating this process, Pasteur removed the microbe's virulence. He attenuated the cholera pathogen, anthrax, and rabies, and he was the first person to develop a rabies vaccine.

Natural Immunization

Natural immunization causes no controversy. Even if it did, there would be nothing anyone could do about it. Natural immunization is a passive form of getting antibodies, meaning someone else gives you preformed antibodies that begin at once to protect you against infection. Your immune system does not need to work at all to get this benefit.

During the third trimester of gestation, IgG antibodies made by the mother go through the placenta into the fetus's bloodstream. These maternal antibodies stay active in the newborn for only about a few weeks to four months. But while they are active, they protect against bacterial and viral infections the same way that IgG protects adults. After their period of activity, these antibodies break down and disappear from the newborn's bloodstream.

At the same time that the maternal IgG is declining, a baby nursing on breast milk gets a second dose of antibodies from Mom. This time they are mainly IgA antibodies, but IgM, IgD, IgG, and IgE are all found in breast milk in small amounts. These antibodies go straight into the baby's digestive tract, where they protect against potential bacterial and viral infections.

Infections in History

British physician Edward Jenner entered medical history in the mid-1800s when he developed the first smallpox vaccine. The first daring experiment with smallpox preceded Jenner, however, when in 1717 Lady Mary Wortley Montagu, wife of Britain's ambassador to Turkey, inoculated her own children with the virus.

Montagu and her brother had suffered with smallpox when they were young—her brother died. Sensing that people who survived smallpox never seemed to get the disease again, Montagu made her children swallow a small specimen taken from the pox scars of an infected person. Montagu's crude experiment worked; her children did not contract smallpox. The technique became known as variolation, named for the variolous matter that pox sores emitted.

Jenner continued developing vaccines safer than those used in variolation. He concentrated mainly on the cowpox virus, which is similar to smallpox. Later, Louis Pasteur coined the term *vaccination* from the Latin *vacca* for "cow" out of respect for Jenner's work on developing safe vaccines.

Babies take in numerous microbes from the things they touch and swallow. Many of the ingested bacteria become part of the good flora that lives with the youngster for life. If an occasional rogue pathogen also lands in the baby's stomach, the battery of antibodies are ready to destroy it or prevent it from passing through the intestinal portal of entry. As an added benefit, Mom has the antibodies needed to fight the microbes most likely to be in her and the baby's immediate surroundings. Breast milk antibodies are therefore fairly specific for particular infections. Because of the preprogramming the immune system does to recognize its own normal flora, the milk antibodies leave the good microbes unharmed.

The protection from milk's antibodies lasts long enough for the baby to begin developing a rudimentary immune system. Recall that this protection is good but not perfect; the very young are considered a high-risk group for infection because of a weak immune system compared to healthy adults.

Infection Vocabulary

Antibodies occupy the serum portion of blood. Serum is blood minus the red blood cells, and it carries oxygen to tissues and platelets, which clots the blood. Since this fluid is loaded with antibodies, medical professionals refer to it as antiserum.

Vaccination and Vaccines

Vaccination is the act of providing immunity by injecting either antigen or antibody directly into a body. A vaccine is the liquid injected into a body that gives it immunity against a specific pathogen. (A small number of vaccines can be taken by swallowing a pill.) Vaccination is an artificial way of getting immunity as opposed to the natural way of receiving antibodies from your mother or building them on your own during infection.

Vaccines can be divided into two types: active or passive. Active vaccines contain an antigen made from a pathogen. When antigen-containing vaccines are put into your body, they force you to make the antibodies against that antigen. Thus you are taking an active part in building your immunity. The passive type contains preformed antibodies. They protect you against infection without any added work from you.

Types of Vaccines

Companies that develop and manufacture vaccines have several ways to put the strongest infection-fighting power into their drug. As a consequence of their research, different vaccines come in any of the following main types:

➤ Live: A vaccine containing living microbes or an active virus

➤ Killed: A vaccine containing an infectious agent that has been completely inactivated

➤ Attenuated: A vaccine containing an infectious agent that has been partially inactivated by removing its virulence, or disease-causing capability, but may still be alive

➤ Macromolecule (also called subunit vaccine): A vaccine made from large molecules derived from an infectious agent but without the agent itself

➤ Conjugated: A vaccine containing more than one component, such as part of a pathogen plus a toxoid

➤ Toxoid: A vaccine made from inactivated toxin

➤ Recombinant: A vaccine made from a microbe that has been genetically engineered to produce an antigen

➤ DNA: A vaccine containing a substance that induces the body's immune system to stimulate antibody production, immune cells, or both

Infection Vocabulary

Genetic engineering is a scientific method in which genetic material from one organism is inserted into the DNA of a second organism. The second organism thus acquires the ability to produce a particular desired end product. DNA vaccines that rely on this technology are now in clinical testing trials for treating several different infectious and noninfectious diseases.

Today's Vaccines

Today, the most common vaccines can be put into two categories: childhood vaccines and adult vaccines. Childhood vaccines include about eleven vaccinations recommended by the CDC to be completed by the time a child is six years old. Health care professionals follow a schedule for giving these vaccinations to children. Also included in childhood vaccines is an additional group of vaccines or boosters recommended for adolescents between seven and eighteen years old.

Following are the childhood vaccines for ages one month through six years (terms in parentheses are the common abbreviations used by health care professionals for these vaccines):

➤ Hepatitis B (HepB)

➤ Rotavirus (RV)

➤ Diphtheria

➤ Tetanus and pertussis (DTaP)

➤ Haemophilus influenzae type b (Hib)

➤ Pneumonococcal pneumonia (PCV)

➤ Poliovirus (IPV)

➤ Influenza

➤ Measles

➤ Mumps and rubella (MMR)

➤ Varicella virus

➤ Hepatitis A (HepA)

➤ Meningitis (MCV4)

Following are the adolescent vaccines for ages seven through eighteen years:

➤ DTaP booster

➤ Human papillomavirus (HPV)

➤ MCV4 booster

➤ Influenza

➤ Pneumococcal pneumonia (under certain conditions)

➤ HepA (under certain conditions)

➤ HepB

➤ IPV

➤ MMR

➤ Varicella

Some of the vaccines on this list are catch-up vaccinations. Catch-up vaccinations are prescribed by doctors for children whose regular vaccination schedule has been delayed.

Adults may get vaccines depending on where they live, a travel destination, or their occupation. These vaccines have no particular schedule and may be given when needed after consulting with a doctor. The most common as-needed vaccines are for the following diseases:

➤ Anthrax

➤ Cholera

➤ Encephalitis

➤ Lyme disease

➤ Plague

➤ Rabies

➤ Shingles

➤ Smallpox

➤ Tuberculosis

➤ Typhoid fever

➤ Typhus

➤ Yellow fever

The influenza vaccine (flu shot) also provides immunity against disease but must be repeated yearly for each new season's prevalent flu strains.

Infection Vocabulary

A booster shot is an additional dose of vaccine given after the initial vaccination. Doctors try to immunize children as early as possible to give them the greatest protection against infection. At early ages, however, maternal antibodies might still be circulating in the child's blood. These antibodies could attack the vaccine just as they attack a real infection. For this reason, the doctor prescribes a booster to ensure that the child gets full protection.

Boosters are usually given a few months to a few years after the initial vaccination. This gives enough time for the antibodies that arose after the initial vaccination to subside so they don't destroy the booster vaccine.

Childhood Vaccines

The following list provides a handy reference for the major childhood vaccines:

➤ HepB: Usually given to newborns within twelve hours of birth. The initial dose, called HepB-1, depends on the mother's exposure to hepatitis B virus. A booster (HepB-2) is given between one and two months of age, and a second booster (HepB-3) comes at six to eighteen months of age. A catch-up HepB series of vaccinations can begin as early as seven years of age and continue to adulthood. All health care workers should be vaccinated against hepatitis B.

➤ RV: This oral vaccine starts no sooner than six weeks of age and is usually given in three doses at two, three, and four months of age. (One manufacturer offers a two-dose vaccine for months two and four only.) Children older than fifteen weeks should not receive this vaccine. The vaccine protects against a common cause of childhood diarrhea.

➤ DTaP: Given in four doses beginning no sooner than six weeks of age. This vaccine contains toxoids of the bacteria *Corynebacterium diphtheriae* (diphtheria) and *Clostridium tetani* (tetanus) and macromolecules from bacterium *Bordetella pertussis* (whooping cough). Tetanus and diphtheria vaccinations should be repeated at ten-year intervals into adulthood.

➤ HiB: This conjugated vaccine protects against the bacterium *Haemophilus influenzae*, one of many causes of pneumonia. Vaccination requires four doses at two, four, and six months of age, with the fourth dose given between twelve to fifteen months of age.

➤ PCV: This vaccine protects against pneumonia caused by about two dozen species of bacteria called pneumococci. This conjugated vaccine is made from parts of various species. Vaccination begins no sooner than six weeks of age in four doses following the same schedule as HiB. This vaccine can also be given to adolescents and adults as needed.

➤ IPV: IPV stands for inactivated poliovirus vaccine. The schedule includes at least four doses beginning no sooner than six weeks, but usually given at two and four months, sometime between six and eighteen months, and between four and six years of age. IPV can also be given in a catch-up schedule. This vaccine used to be given as a pill until the year 2000. The oral form had been shown to cause about nine cases of polio annually. This risk has been eliminated by using injected vaccine.

➤ MMR: The MMR vaccine protects against the viruses rubeola (measles), mumps, and German measles (rubella). The vaccine is made from live viruses that have been attenuated to eliminate their ability to cause illness. The first dose occurs between twelve and fifteen months of age, and a booster is given between ages four and six years. A catch-up schedule is available for MMR.

➤ Varicella: This vaccine protects against the virus of the same name, the cause of chickenpox and shingles. The vaccination schedule is the same as for MMR, and a catch-up schedule is available. Children who have not had chickenpox can be vaccinated at about ages eleven to twelve years to prevent adult chickenpox. At age thirteen years or older, a person can receive a two-dose vaccination no less than four weeks apart.

➤ HepA: The HepA vaccine protects against hepatitis A virus infection. This vaccine is administered in children twelve months or older in two doses at least six months apart. This vaccine is also recommended for any adolescent or adult traveling to areas where hepatitis A is common. Other high-risk groups that should consider vaccination against hepatitis A are health care workers, intravenous drug users, homosexual men, and people with chronic liver diseases.

➤ MCV4: This abbreviation stands for meningococcal conjugate vaccine, quadrivalent. The word *quadrivalent* means the vaccine contains four distinct parts from various bacteria known to cause the disease meningitis. Not every child needs MCV4 vaccination. In parts of the world where meningitis is common, vaccination may begin when a child is two to four years old. Other children can wait until age eleven or twelve, or use a catch-up schedule if they are thirteen years or older. The vaccine is given in two doses at least eight weeks apart.

In the first six years of life, a kid gets a lot of vaccines! Drug companies have worked hard to invent vaccines compatible with each other so that more than one can be given in the same shot. These so-called combination vaccines are available for HepB plus Hib and for DTaP, IPV, and HepB.

At the Doctor's Office

In the 1980s and 1990s, parents began skipping some of the vaccinations recommended for their children. The reasons for this decision varied, but they often related to concerns over vaccine safety or the mistaken belief that many childhood diseases had been eliminated from society. Sometimes a child's vaccination records are incomplete and a doctor has no way of knowing which vaccinations have been given and which are missing. In other instances, a vaccination schedule was disrupted. As a result, the CDC devised a schedule for catching up with childhood vaccinations in older children. Catch-up vaccination schedules are tailored to the child's known history of vaccinations. Your doctor can help you determine what shots are needed for your child and when.

The Flu Vaccine

The flu shot is a yearly vaccine that can be given to children as young as six months and can be continued into late adulthood. The composition of these vaccines varies from year to year. This variation occurs because each year scientists try to predict which two or three strains of the flu will be the most troublesome in the coming flu season. But they must make these predictions by testing samples from animals during the previous year. This gives time for vaccine manufacturers to produce a yearly batch of vaccines. Some years the flu vaccine contains antigens for the very same strains that emerge in our population in November. In those years, the flu shot becomes an effective deterrent to the spread of influenza. Other years, well, they get it wrong. In those years, the flu shot seems to be less effective against the flu.

The CDC recommends that you always get a seasonal flu shot even if the year's strains do not match exactly with the vaccine's strains. In this circumstance, the vaccine might reduce the severity of the infection if you catch the flu.

The flu vaccine is made from influenza strains that have been killed by exposure to a chemical. But they are still antigens, and the body reacts to them as such. These reactions show up as side effects, mainly soreness at the injection site, fever, body aches, and sore throat.

Microbe Basics

Tiny spikes on the outside of the influenza virus determine how the flu changes from season to season. The virus uses these spikes to attach to mucous membranes in your nose and throat, and they can change from year to year.

Two types of spikes exist, both made of glycoprotein. H spikes number about five hundred all over the virus surface. These spikes help the virus recognize mucous membrane tissue. N spikes total only about one hundred and the virus uses them to spread from cell to cell in the respiratory tract.

Virologists identify flu viruses based on the type of H and N spikes they find after analyzing the virus. The flu virus is therefore named H1, H2, H3, and so on plus N1, N2, N3, and so on. The result is a flu called H1N1 or other derivations.

Rabies Vaccination

People who have a high risk of being exposed to the rabies virus receive this vaccine. For example, veterinarians, animal care technicians, zoo employees, and wildlife handlers should consider getting vaccinated. The most common animal carriers of the rabies virus are bats, raccoons, skunks, coyotes, foxes, dogs, and cats. If you're thinking of taking up spelunking as a serious hobby, get a rabies vaccination. The virus can be spread by bats by bites and by inhalation of virus-containing droplets inside caves with dense bat populations.

The rabies vaccine is made from active viruses that have been inactivated in a laboratory. People working in these production laboratories should also receive the vaccine.

Vaccination against rabies requires three doses. The first two are separated by seven days and the third dose follows the second by twenty-one days.

Cholera Vaccination

The cholera vaccination is another vaccine people should consider only under special circumstances. It is needed for those traveling to places where the cholera disease is a recurring problem. Cholera comes from ingesting water that has been contaminated by *Vibrio cholerae* bacteria. Areas that experience frequent flooding combined with poor sanitation and faulty infrastructure for drinking water and sewage should raise a red flag in your mind.

The cholera vaccine comes from whole bacteria cells that have been treated to remove their virulence. These types of vaccines tend to be less effective than others. For example, the cholera vaccine does not assure 100 percent protection from infection. Also, the protection lasts for only three to six months.

Shingles Vaccination

Shingles is a painful rash prominent on certain parts of the body lasting for up to four weeks. Caused by the varicella zoster virus, this rash flares up periodically over several years. The rash usually breaks out on the scalp, neck, and shoulders, and across the ribs. This illness is a latent disease that follows a chickenpox infection. Several decades can intervene before shingles appears in a person who had once been infected with the chickenpox virus.

The vaccine against shingles appeared on the market in the United States in 2006. It cannot ensure 100 percent protection from shingles. The vaccine can, however, lessen the symptoms of shingles and may prevent it altogether in some people.

Most doctors recommend that if you decide to get this vaccine, you get it at about age sixty.

Herd Immunity

Herd immunity is a phenomenon in which a pathogen fails to spread through a population because most of the people are immune. It works like this: Say you have a population of 1,000 people, 900 of whom have immunity against pathogen A. Their immunity can come from natural immunity or from vaccination. To keep the infection going, the pathogen must find a susceptible host. In other words, pathogen A must find the one susceptible host for every ten people. Statistically, this gives the entire population, the herd, a pretty good chance of staying uninfected.

Opponents of vaccination programs, such as those recommended for children, often use herd immunity as a reason for not having their children vaccinated. These parents feel that herd immunity will protect their children. Of course, that approach can only work if most people cooperate with recommended vaccination programs. If most people decided to opt out, herd immunity would crash and pathogens would find many more susceptible people

Infection Vocabulary

A mass vaccination is a concerted program carried out in many countries to vaccinate their residents against a certain disease. The most successful mass vaccination program ever conducted occurred between 1950 and 1979, when smallpox was eradicated worldwide.

to infect. In herd immunity, the strength of a group is greater than its individual parts.

Vaccine Safety

In the earliest days of vaccine development, scientists experimenting with vaccines often contracted the very disease they were trying to prevent. This occurrence has long disappeared from current practices, but many people still view vaccines with skepticism.

The MMR has received the most vehement opposition by people convinced that it causes autism in children. Autism is a developmental condition in which a child withdraws from normal communication with others and may resort to primitive or repetitive behavior. Autism symptoms tend to appear about the same time children are getting many of their childhood vaccinations. This has led many people to conclude there is a cause and effect. In fact, many studies on the causes of autism have failed to build an unarguable link between the vaccines and the condition.

Vaccines are like any drug: there will be side effects. A drug is a substance put into the body with the intent of changing the body's normal workings. Extremely rare is the drug that can complete its intended task without interfering with some other process in the body.

Consider this, however: Hundreds of thousands of vaccines are given around the world every year. The number of people becoming gravely ill from a vaccine is infinitesimally small compared to the millions who die each year from preventable infectious disease—deaths because no vaccines were available to them.

Vaccine Side Effects

Excluding the very rare instances of serious side effects, vaccines can give some mild discomfort. These symptoms usually last for no more than a few days. Here are some of the typical side effects seen in many of the vaccines discussed in this chapter:

➤ Soreness, redness, or swelling at the injection site

➤ Fever

➤ Irritability

➤ Body aches

➤ Hoarseness or sore throat

➤ Mild rash

➤ Drowsiness or tiredness

At the Doctor's Office

Gene therapy is a promising new avenue in disease treatment that uses the principles of vaccination. In gene therapy, a bioengineer puts a therapeutic gene into an attenuated virus. (A therapeutic gene is any gene that helps correct a medical problem in the body.) The virus is then injected into the body like a vaccine. The virus then finds its target tissue, infects the cells, and inserts the therapeutic gene into the host's DNA.

The Consequences of Not Immunizing

We have done such a good job of ridding certain pathogens from our communities that many people believe the threat from pathogens no longer exists. Combined with inaccurate information on the safety of vaccines, many parents now skip having their children vaccinated. They also bypass any adult vaccines for themselves.

Refusing to follow an accepted vaccination program for you or your family will not make you healthier. Failure to immunize has created a reemergence of many diseases that were once very rare. Meningitis, whooping cough, measles, and chickenpox are now considered reemerging diseases because of parents' past decision to skip immunizations for their children. In a few instances, doctors have been to blame for the lax attitude toward immunizing because they have never seen a case of measles in their career. The success of vaccination programs has lulled people into a false sense that the danger is gone.

Vaccination is like other medical topics in that you are best served by seeking reputable resources to learn more about the subject and telling your doctor of the specific questions you have about vaccine safety. Medical researchers uncover new details about vaccination, infection, and immunity every year. Therefore, the information changes, and it is every adult's responsibility to learn as much as they can for making sound decisions about their health.

PART FIVE

Specialized Infections

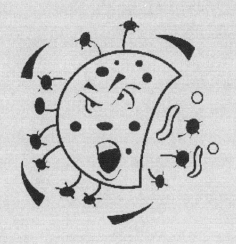

CHAPTER 22

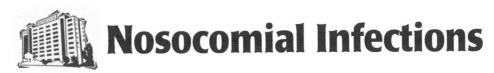 # Nosocomial Infections

In This Chapter

➤ Why hospitals have lots of germs

➤ What you can and cannot control when fighting hospital germs

➤ How hospitals prevent infection in patients

➤ The basics of antiseptics

➤ The main pathogens that cause nosocomial infections

In this chapter you will learn what to do about hospital germs. The hospital is "crawling" with germs mainly because this is a place where a lot of sick people congregate. But other factors contribute to nosocomial, or hospital-derived, infections. Although we blame hospitals for much of the trouble with germs, keep in mind this chapter applies to additional facilities such as doctors' and dentists' offices, outpatient clinics, and nursing homes.

Why Hospitals Have So Many Germs

Hospitals carry germs for the obvious reason that they are places where lots of sick people reside. Infectious agents that move by way of direct and indirect contact and droplet transmission also find more susceptible hosts in densely packed populations than in groups where people are spread out. In this way a hospital resembles a college dorm, a military base, and a sports team's locker room.

Hospitals and other places where health care professionals tend to patients also possess certain characteristics that help germs move around. See if you can figure out how these characteristics of hospitals contribute to germ transmission:

➤ Patient populations with underlying disease, chronic health problems, or immunocompromised status

➤ A high incidence in the patient population of open wounds, burns, or surgical incision sites

➤ Health care providers who move from patient to patient to assess health and make observations

➤ Health care providers who touch patients by helping them get into and out of bed, use bathrooms and showers, use bedpans, give sponge baths or massages, and change bedding

➤ Medical instruments that are used in or on a patient's body

➤ Food prepared at a centrally located kitchen, then delivered by cart to patient rooms

For health care workers to break the chain of transmission, hygiene is essential. This includes not only personal hygiene by healthcare professionals, but also hospital hygiene. By this, I mean a hospital must have a strong sanitation program to help block germ transmission.

Infection Vocabulary

The word *nosocomial* comes from two Greek roots, "noso" and "komos." *Noso* refers to any situation involving disease. The root *komos* refers to a person who attends to the sick. The English language version of the combined words results in nosocomial, which pertains to hospitals and infirmaries.

Things You Cannot Control in a Hospital

If you spend any time during your life as a hospital patient, you will be at the mercy of things related to your health that you cannot control. You have no way of knowing if your surgeon scrubbed up properly before your surgery, or if the food tray was in the hallway for an extra thirty minutes before arriving at your room, or if that nurse who just took your temperature forgot to wash his hands after checking on Mr. P in the next room. If the hand washing was forgotten, you'd better hope Mr. P isn't the guy keeping you up all night with a hacking cough!

Be aware of the sanitary conditions around you in a hospital. It's okay to ask the nurse, or a worker delivering meals, books, magazines, and water pitchers, if she washed her hands.

Keep an eagle eye out for dirty or blood-splattered uniforms worn by health care workers just as you would note a slovenly waitperson in a restaurant. Unfortunately, you can walk out of a restaurant that makes you uneasy; you cannot walk out of a hospital. You can, however, ask a worker to wash his or her hands before tending to you. Beware of workers wearing fake nails, chewing gum, or sporting a beard. Note the cleaning crew workers. Are they doing a good job of cleaning the entire floor, or do they use a mop that looks like World War II surplus and filthy cleaning solution that may be even older?

Hospitals have worked hard to improve their record of spreading nosocomial infections. For many years, at least 5 to 10 percent of all hospital patients acquired some nosocomial infection with their hospital stay. The risks increased the longer patients stayed in the hospital. Now the infection rate may be as low as 2 patients infected per 1,000.

This improvement came partly from studies run by microbiologists showing that hospital workers had been remiss in good personal hygiene. About half of all nurses and doctors did not wash their hands properly or at all between seeing patients or after using the restroom!

Never be afraid to speak up if your instincts tell you the cleanliness of your hospital room or care is iffy. If you are not in condition to voice your concerns, have an advocate speak up for you.

Things You Can Control in a Hospital

Start blocking germ transmission by washing your hands before eating, after using the bathroom or a bedpan, and by doing anything else that adds up to good personal hygiene. Hospitals have begun supplying patients with alcohol-based hand sanitizers. A dispenser of similar product usually exists somewhere in the hallways. Use these products and ask your visitors to do so as well. Consider also these precautions:

➤ After surgery, use a spirometer as often as your nurse recommends. This device helps strengthen your lungs and so reduces your risk of catching pneumonia.

➤ If you have had a catheter inserted, ask that it be removed at the earliest possible moment. Remind nurses to check on your catheter for possible clogging. If you feel any pain, speak up immediately.

➤ Ask your nurse if your intravenous (IV) line is being checked often for signs of clogging. Pay attention to the site where your IV fluid enters your body. Report any pain or swelling immediately.

➤ Reject any meal that arrives with the food left uncovered, beverage containers open, dirty silverware, or any other signs of dirt or filth.

➤ Make sure your nurse wears disposable gloves when touching your mucous membranes or body secretions. If the nurse doesn't take this precaution with you, how can you be sure he or she did the same with the previous patient?

➤ Don't depend on antibiotics to save you. Antibiotics are a last resort in fighting infection, and they are losing their effectiveness by the day as antibiotic-resistant microbes increase. Hospitals have particularly high incidence rates of antibiotic-resistant pathogens.

Microbe Basics

Pseudomonas aeruginosa is a ubiquitous microbe, meaning it lives just about everywhere. This species of bacteria can be found on plants, in soil, and in water. The *P. aeruginosa* in water presents an especially high risk of infection in hospitals because it gets into the body with any fluid. Nosocomial infections started by *P. aeruginosa* are associated most with the following:

➤ Urinary tract infections from contaminated catheters

➤ Infected skin from contaminated bandaging of burn wounds

➤ Sepsis from contaminated IV fluids

➤ Pneumonia from prolonged use of devices inserted in the respiratory tract

The Basics of Antiseptics

Antiseptics play a crucial role in reducing germ transmission in hospitals. An antiseptic is any substance that removes microbes from your skin. The use of an antiseptic is therefore critical to preventing infection when used just prior to giving you a shot or making an incision. Health care workers might also clean your skin with an antiseptic before putting an external instrument on your body, such as the sensors connected to an electrocardiograph.

Antiseptics remove any pathogens that might be on your skin and reduce the numbers of normal flora, which could enter your body to cause an opportunistic infection. Antiseptics do not sterilize the skin; some microbes always remain attached tightly to skin. Antiseptic use, however, greatly reduces the likelihood of infection. The few normal flora that gets through your skin can be eliminated by your immune system and the antibiotics you'll probably receive while being a hospital patient.

A variety of antiseptic products work equally well in protecting patients from infection. Some of these chemicals may sound familiar to you; others may not:

➤ Acridines: Mainly acriflavine and aminoacridine

➤ Alcohols: Mainly isopropyl alcohol and water-free, alcohol-based sanitizers, but also ethanol and benzyl alcohol

➤ Chlorines: Mainly chlorhexidine and solutions containing chloramine

➤ Iodine: Formulas called tincture of iodine and iodophor

➤ Peroxides: Mainly hydrogen peroxide, benzoyl peroxide, and peracetic acid

➤ Phenols, sometimes called carbolic acid: These are phenol, bisphenol, and triclosan

➤ Quats, short for quaternary ammonium compounds: The most common is benzalkonium chloride

➤ Salicylic compounds: Includes salicylic acid and salicylamide

Of the antiseptics listed above, the alcohols, chlorines, quats, and peroxides may be most common in health care. Beware that health care workers sometimes refer to these solutions as disinfectants. It's a fine distinction, but the word *disinfectant* applies more accurately to chemicals for removing germs from only inanimate surfaces (see Chapter 12).

At the Doctor's Office

Rubbing alcohol may also be labeled as isopropyl alcohol. Some manufacturers help you by calling it isopropyl rubbing alcohol. By any name, rubbing alcohol works best in killing germs when used as a 70 percent solution with water. At this concentration, the alcohol level is high enough to kill microbial cells, but the water keeps it from evaporating too quickly. If pure alcohol were used, it would evaporate in a few seconds and might not be in contact with the microbes long enough to affect them.

You don't have to dilute alcohol in water when you get home after buying it. Rubbing alcohol sold in pharmacies and grocery stores is already set to 70 percent. But check to be sure.

In hospitals, doctors' and dentists' offices, and other places where patients go for treatment, antiseptics are used mainly for the following tasks:

➤ Hand washing between patient visits

➤ Skin preparation before giving an injection or making a surgical incision

➤ Presurgery hand scrubbing

Surgery

The surgery room is a place where health care workers apply the best lessons they've learned about hygiene, sanitation, antiseptics, disinfection, and sterilization. A well-trained surgeon and support staff will keep germs away from the patient during surgery and will watch out for trouble following surgery. All of the following components go into action for preventing infections associated with a surgery of any type:

➤ Disinfection of the surgery room, including floor and walls, and use of a special filter in the ventilation system to prevent the entry of microbes

➤ Sterilization, removal of all living matter, of surgical instruments

➤ Preoperative dose of antibiotics to protect the patient from any microbe that dares get into the body

➤ Preoperative scrubbing by surgeons and support personnel to assure their hands and arms contain no pathogens

➤ Preoperative "gowning" in sterile gloves, gown, mask, hat, and booties to prevent any normal flora from the surgeon from coming in contact with the patient

➤ Use of antiseptic on the patient's skin prior to making a surgical incision or insertion of an IV needle

➤ Postoperative dose of antibiotics as insurance against infection

All of these activities are intended to prevent septicemia, sepsis, and local infections at the surgical incision and IV sites.

Despite the efforts to prevent nosocomial infections, they continue to occur in every hospital. The most common are urinary tract infections (UTIs), lower respiratory tract infections (mainly pneumonia), and septicemia. A smaller portion of nosocomial events may show up also as skin infections and local infections at a surgical incision site. After getting out of surgery, you may feel lousy, but do your best to pay attention to your body. Look for pain, swelling, redness, or other signs of infection.

Infections and Disease

Septicemia is the presence of a microbe in the blood. This potentially serious situation can occur in hospital patients because of the use of needles and IV lines, and open wounds. A strong immune system helps fight septicemia. Hospital patients also receive antibiotics during their stay, which help reduce the chance of these infections.

Sepsis is a more serious condition in which pathogens have entered the bloodstream and some organs or tissues. The entire body reacts with inflammation and fever. Various organs can be stressed during sepsis because of poor blood flow associated with abnormal heart rate and breathing. Organ failure, shock, and death can occur if sepsis is not swiftly arrested.

The Major Nosocomial Pathogens

The pathogens that start most nosocomial infections also are capable of causing illness outside of a hospital. No magic pathogen is known to exist only in hospitals, but hospitals do carry their own brand of normal flora. Hospital flora can be as distinctive for a given hospital as they are for individuals.

Years of study have shown these microbes to show up time and again in nosocomial infections:

➤ *Pseudomonas aeruginosa*: Found in many infections perhaps because it is common indoors and outside. *P. aeruginosa* is a major participant in UTIs, infections in burn victims, septicemia, and nosocomial pneumonias. This bacterium exists in almost all forms of water, including tap, bottled, and purified water.

➤ *Clostridium difficile*: A common cause of diarrhea in infants, this bacterium is capable of wiping out the normal flora of the intestines. Sometimes, its growth is aided by antibiotics that remove the normal flora and let resistant *C. difficile* take over the body.

➤ *Staph aureus*: This bacterium shows up in skin wounds, incision sites, the lower respiratory tract, and in septicemia. Various antibiotic-resistant strains, mainly MRSA, may have originated in hospitals, where antibiotic use is widespread.

➤ *Enterococci*: Various species of enteric (from the intestines) bacteria. Often from fecal contamination, these bacteria spread from patient to patient through direct contact and are carried by hospital workers. These bacteria cause UTIs, lower respiratory tract infections, septicemia, skin infections, and infections at surgical incision sites. The antibiotic-resistant strain called VRE belongs to this group.

➤ *Enterobacter* species: These bacteria are also from intestines. They differ from the enterococci by being shaped like a rod rather than spherical.

➤ *E. coli*: Wherever there's infection, you cannot overlook *E. coli* as a possible perpetrator. This bacterium lives only in the intestines and yet it seems to be everywhere when microbiologists go on the hunt for germ hot spots. *E. coli* has been found in UTIs, skin infections, surgical wounds, and as a cause of food-borne illness.

➤ *Candida albicans*: This yeast always poses a threat when people take antibiotics. The antibiotics reduce the numbers of normal flora on the body, and *Candida* then grows to larger-than-normal numbers on the body. *Candida* has been found in UTIs and in cases of septicemia.

Microbe Basics

Clostridium difficile belongs to the same genus as the bacteria that cause botulism toxicity, tetanus, and gangrene. This species, however, focuses mainly on the digestive tract of people who have been receiving antibiotics. The result of *C. difficile* infection is watery diarrhea that is usually foul smelling and may contain mucus or blood. Other symptoms include fever and abdominal cramping.

C. difficile causes particular problems in infants and young children who are hospitalized. One reason for its success as a nosocomial pathogen relates to its ability to make spores. The rugged endospore form of all clostridia resists chemicals, heating, drying, and nutrient deprivation. These bacteria, therefore, withstand many of the challenges that other bacteria cannot.

Visiting a Hospital Patient

When you visit a patient who's in the hospital, you can protect your health and the patient's by following this advice:

➤ Don't visit at all if you are sick with a cold, the flu, or any other condition that has weakened your immunity.

➤ Avoid touching things the entire time you are visiting a patient.

➤ Use your own pen to sign in at the front desk. Don't share the patient's drinking cup, and avoid flipping through the shared magazines in the waiting area.

➤ Wearing a mask isn't necessary when visiting the sick—it sends an undeniable message of doom—but try not to cough, sneeze, laugh, or even talk animatedly in the patient's face.

➤ Wash your hands at the appropriate times to maintain good personal hygiene, but also wash them after leaving the hospital at the end of your visit. Use the hand sanitizer dispensers that dot most hospital hallways these days.

Nosocomial infections are a little like food-borne illness. Sometimes even your best efforts appear hopeless against a pathogen determined to enter your body. Hospitals and restaurants also employ a large staff with varied hygiene habits despite the best training their supervisors try to instill.

The best tips for fighting nosocomial infections and avoiding spreading them to others go back to the principles of good personal hygiene. But be on the lookout as you would in any restaurant for something that looks suspicious. Report it, avoid it, or do whatever it takes to make the hospital a place safe from germ transmission.

CHAPTER 23

Emerging and Reemerging Infectious Diseases

In This Chapter

➤ The hallmarks of emerging and reemerging diseases

➤ The reasons for today's new emerging diseases

➤ The main emerging diseases and the responsible pathogens

➤ Tips for keeping track of emerging diseases

This chapter covers emerging infectious diseases. These are diseases that appear (or are documented) in the population for the first time.

The subject of emerging infectious diseases usually includes a subcategory called reemerging diseases. Reemerging infectious diseases are those that were thought to have disappeared from a population but have returned. Sometimes epidemiologists may have a hard time telling them apart. They need to decide if the disease just emerged for the first time or if it had existed undetected before. In truth, the list of emerging diseases probably contains both types.

Any discussion on emerging infectious diseases must include the zoonotic diseases. These diseases come from animal populations before they emerge in human populations. In this chapter you will see how people's relationship with the environment affects the animal carriers that harbor many human diseases. If emerging diseases are on the rise, so too are zoonotic diseases.

Emerging and Reemerging

The last known case of smallpox was eradicated in Somalia in 1977. A few years later, the World Health Assembly declared the world officially free of smallpox. The combination of medical perseverance and vaccination hinted that other ancient infectious diseases would finally disappear. But besides smallpox, no other infectious disease has disappeared. On the contrary, new pathogens emerge every few years to startle the medical community and put it in defensive mode.

Microbe Basics

Smallpox virus causes an acute, contagious, and systemic (throughout the body) disease. Its symptoms are skin eruptions that pass through several stages of bumps or pimples (papules), blisters (vesicles), pustules (pimples filled with white blood cells), and crusts.

Smallpox has been eradicated from the world population. Specimens of the virus are stored in a small number of research laboratories.

We know now that complex factors interrelate to cause a disease to emerge or reemerge. Emergence is largely due to changes in human behavior that affect disease patterns in a population. Environmental factors also play a part. Sometimes a disease emerges or disappears for no apparent reason. In time, researchers usually determine the cause of a disease's emergence or disappearance, but the mystery can last years or decades before the pieces finally fall together. Consider the following three examples of emergence: AIDS, hantavirus, and the bubonic plague.

The AIDS Epidemic

In 1980, a variety of rare infections were being reported by doctors caring for patients who were homosexual men. The infections attacked almost every system in the body, causing everything from superficial skin infections to nervous system disorders. The doctors also noticed the infections were being caused by bacteria, fungi, protozoa, and viruses that seldom caused problems in their other patients. It was eventually discovered that the infections were secondary to the main cause of the growing epidemic, the AIDS virus.

AIDS offers an example of an emerging disease: it came seemingly from out of nowhere. The transmission of the AIDS virus was attributable in part to a change in social behavior in the two decades prior to its emergence. Infecting first homosexual men and intravenous drug users, the virus infected a few people, and then spread into an increasingly large subpopulation.

Hantavirus Infection

Hantavirus emerged in 1993 in the southwestern United States. The virus causes a pulmonary syndrome characterized by edema (fluid accumulation) in the lungs. Since then, virologists have identified the Sin Nombre strain of hantavirus as the main pathogen in the United States. Other hantavirus strains have caused infections elsewhere in the world.

Hantavirus is carried by rodents, mainly deer mice, native to deserts of the U.S. Southwest. Transmission is likely from inhaling particles from dried rodent feces. Why did this virus emerge in the early 1990s? The rapid growth of housing developments during this period encroached into desert lands that had laid undisturbed forever—until then. In a few years, people were living in places that put them in proximity to the virus's reservoir. The hantavirus outbreak became an example of a combination of changing human behavior and environmental factors.

Bubonic Plague

The plague periodically emerges in localized areas of the world. This disease is caused the bacterium *Yersinia pestis*, which is carried by rodents such as rats.

Plague epidemics have ravaged societies from earliest recorded history to the seventeenth century. After that time, plague outbreaks became rare. The reasons for the plague's disappearance are only partially known. Undoubtedly, a stronger commitment to community sanitation and hygiene helped drive the pathogen back to its reservoir.

Infections and Disease

The World Health Organization (WHO) is the global health arm of the United Nations. The WHO's website and publications provide the best resources for global health issues and the main infectious disease threats worldwide. The WHO also provides updates on outbreaks of emerging infectious diseases.

Yet plague outbreaks continue today. Since 2001, plague outbreaks have occurred yearly, mainly in Asia, Africa, and South America. This zoonotic disease is linked to dense rat populations. Therefore, its periodic emergence almost always relates to rising poverty in the affected area.

The Reasons for Today's Emerging Diseases

It's difficult to find just one reason for an infection to emerge. More often, many complex reasons intertwine. In the list of reasons for emergence and reemergence of infectious disease, notice how many relate to changing patterns in human populations, such as where people live, the distances they travel, and how urban areas change:

➤ Climate change: This is a controversial subject that has not yet been fully defined. Epidemiologists nonetheless predict changes in infectious disease emergence because of climate change-induced events. Warmer temperatures affect the breeding behavior of animal reservoirs and insect vectors. Temperature also impacts weather patterns. Increased flooding that can be expected to occur with global warming will expand the breeding waters for mosquitoes.

➤ Evolution: Microbes naturally change. Some changes will invariably lead to stronger, more virulent, and perhaps more antibiotic-resistant pathogens.

➤ Food production and distribution: Modern methods of mass producing and distributing food on a global scale can spread food-borne illness farther than ever before.

➤ Globalization: This complex subject includes international business travel, global shipping of goods, and other hallmarks of global commerce. Ships, airplanes, and trains now move pathogens that hitchhike to new countries and regions of the world.

➤ Human behavior: Changing social attitudes influence behavior toward travel, sex, and other means of interacting with each other.

➤ International travel: Pathogens now move faster across the globe than epidemiologists can track them.

➤ Military conflicts: An aspect of politics, military conflicts destroy infrastructure, disrupt clean water supplies and sewage removal, interfere with distribution of medicines, and cause mass migrations of displaced people.

➤ Population growth: Pathogens move into new communities as urban populations expand. New developments also put people in closer contact with wildlife reservoirs and insect and animal vectors.

➤ Poverty: This is a major reason infectious disease will not go away. Hallmarks of poverty are poor nutrition, inadequate shelter, missing healthcare and vaccination programs, no access to clean water, and faulty or no sanitation in communities. All of these factors increase the chance of infection.

An additional environmental change that may affect the patterns of infectious diseases is biodiversity loss. As species go extinct at an alarming rate, other species gain an opportunity to take over new habitats. This shift in the types and numbers of animals, insects, and plants in our future may also influence the patterns of disease.

Infections in History

The increased globalization of business and recreational travel has left few places on Earth free from invasive species. An invasive species is any plant or animal that now thrives in a place different from its natural habitat. Global shipping and travel move microbes around the world. These microbes either travel attached to people, animals, or products, or they are inside insects carried by people, animals, or products. Infectious agents can now spread more swiftly than in any other time in history.

Important Emerging Diseases

Some diseases listed by the WHO as emerging diseases seem like they have been around a long time. Often, the disease retains its emerging status because it is still emerging in new parts of the world.

No time limit exists on how fast a disease must show up in a population to be considered an emerging disease. Some diseases emerge slowly but steadily; others make a sudden appearance.

Important emerging diseases worldwide include some that may seem like reemerging diseases. For example, yellow fever has haunted society for four hundred years, and then it had almost disappeared in the last century. The WHO lists it

Infections and Disease

Five types of hepatitis virus exist: A, B, C, D, and E. Each infects liver tissue, but their modes of transmission are distinctive.

Hepatitis A and E are waterborne and food-borne pathogens. Hepatitis B, C, and D usually transmit via exchange of body fluids; hepatitis B is classified as an STD. Hepatitis B also passes from an infected mother to her child at birth, but this contagious virus may also be transmitted by vehicles and direct nonsexual contact with an infected person.

The risk of infection with hepatitis A and B are high in many large regions of the world. Only the United States, Canada, Western Europe, and Australia are currently low-risk areas.

Hepatitis B and C cause chronic disease and have infected billions of people worldwide. In many of these cases, the infected person has no symptoms. When symptoms occur, they are mainly jaundice, dark urine, fatigue, nausea, and abdominal pain.

as an emerging disease because it is now showing up in new regions. You can also think of yellow fever as a reemerging infectious disease because it had once existed in a population, disappeared, and then returned.

The WHO lists these infectious diseases as emerging:

➤ Anthrax: This bacterial disease caused by *Bacillus anthracis* continues to show up in places dependent on raising livestock andexperiencing a breakdown in livestock vaccination programs.

➤ Crimean-Congo hemorrhagic fever (CCHF): The disease is caused by a tick-borne virus. The infection is increasing in Africa, Asia, the Middle East, and the Balkans.

➤ Dengue fever: Currently, dengue fever is the most common mosquito-borne infection. As many as 2.5 billion people live in areas where they can easily be infected by the virus through a mosquito bite.

➤ Ebola hemorrhagic fever: The Ebola virus causes sporadic outbreaks in African countries every year.

➤ Hendra virus infection: This virus carried by fruit bats affects horses and people. The severe flulike disease is currently experiencing sporadic outbreaks in Australia.

➤ Hepatitis: Five different types of the hepatitis virus infect the liver. Hepatitis causes local outbreaks worldwide.

➤ Influenza: Influenza reemerges every year. Each new strain of avian (bird) flu or swine flu represents an emerging disease. Confusing? Maybe so. Influenza virus remains one of medicine's most confounding enemies and accounts for thousands of deaths worldwide each year.

➤ Lassa fever: This deadly disease caused by the Lassa virus is spread by rodents. The main route of transmission is by vehicles contaminated by rodent feces.

➤ Marburg hemorrhagic fever: This often fatal disease is caused by the Marburg virus. It is currently in epidemic proportions in sub-Saharan Africa.

➤ Meningococcal disease: The bacterium *Neisseria meningitidis* causes this contagious meningitis. It is spread by droplet transmission.

➤ Human monkeypox infection: The monkeypox virus causes a disease similar to smallpox. Outbreaks are concentrated in villages of central and western Africa, but in 2003 the disease occurred in the United States. The U.S. outbreak was thought to have been carried by rodents from Africa that passed the pathogen to prairie dogs in the U.S. Midwest.

➤ Nipah virus infection: The Nipah virus emerged about ten years ago in Malaysia. People and animals are infected when bitten by a fruit bat that carries the pathogen.

➤ Plague: This ancient disease continues to cause outbreaks.

➤ Rift Valley fever: The Rift Valley virus is carried from animals to humans by mosquitoes. Cattle and other livestock are serving as the reservoir for outbreaks, mainly in Africa.

➤ Severe Acute Respiratory Syndrome (SARS): This infection caused by the coronavirus emerged in Asia in 2003. It continues to cause sporadic outbreaks.

➤ Tularemia: This bacterial infection caused by *Francisella tularensis* is transmitted by various routes. Transmission can be by airborne moisture droplets, direct contact with an infected person, or a bite from an infected tick or mosquito. Fewer than ten pathogens may be enough to cause infection.

➤ Yellow fever: The yellow fever virus is transmitted by mosquito bite. The disease is called yellow fever because of the jaundice (yellowing) that occurs in the eyes and skin.

Emerging Zoonotic Diseases (Zoonoses)

Zoonotic disease is an illness communicable from animals (vertebrates only) to humans. More than 250 pathogens are known to begin the infection chain in an animal reservoir. Although an animal can carry any type of pathogen, viruses and bacteria tend to cause most zoonotic diseases.

I will cover zoonotic diseases in more detail in the next chapter. Here, I'll explain why new diseases often emerge from animal populations.

The answer to why there exists a strong emerging disease-animal connection might be found in the changing behaviors between people and animals. I am referring not only to an increased devotion to our pets, but also to an increase in the exotic pets trade, the desire to experience nature by going to wilderness areas, and an interest in environment. Animal reservoirs are widespread and an enlarging human population comes in contact with animals with increasing frequency. Zoonotic diseases can originate in wildlife, domesticated farm animals, and pets. Even service animals assigned to help blind or deaf people have been implicated in zoonotic disease.

In most instances of animal-to-human transmission of infection, an insect vector carries the pathogen. Bites and other types of animal-human interactions are much less common than vector transmission.

Infections and Disease

The coronavirus responsible for Severe Acute Respiratory Syndrome (SARS) causes a severe contagious form of pneumonia with symptoms arising from two to ten days after infection. Like other pneumonias, the pathogen uses droplet transmission and results in typical pneumonia symptoms: persistent cough, mild fever, difficult breathing, and headache and muscle aches. Lungs weakened by SARS often get a secondary pneumonia infection caused by bacteria.

SARS first emerged in 2003 in a businessman who had traveled from his home in Guangdong Province, China, to Vietnam by way of Hong Kong. This forty-eight-year-old man died of the disease as did the doctor who had diagnosed the illness.

Following the initial outbreak, public health agencies have been proactive in preventing further spread of SARS. Recommendations for preventing infection and spread of the SARS coronavirus are the same as for preventing cold and flu viruses: cover up when coughing or sneezing, avoid sharing utensils and food, and use proper hand washing. The use of hand sanitizers and disinfectants as appropriate also blocks SARS transmission.

Coronavirus is a classic zoonotic pathogen. It causes respiratory and digestive tract infections in livestock. Among poultry, coronavirus is especially common in ducks. Like influenza, the virus makes a species-jump to humans in places where people live in proximity to infected animals.

Defenses Against Emerging Disease

You have little control over the emergence of a disease in a faraway land. Most of the time, you can't control a pathogen's migration into your community. The basics of fighting an emerging germ are exactly the same as fighting a pathogen that has been established in a community for a long time. After all, the germ doesn't care whether it is emerging in a population has been there for centuries. Every pathogen must follow the same mantra of infection: encounter a susceptible host, gain entry into the host, find a favorite host tissue, and multiply.

The principles of hygiene, disinfection, and sanitation remain in force for emerging diseases. You can, however, increase your knowledge of diseases as they emerge. By this I mean, know your surroundings. If your life involves no big changes in the near future, your chances of meeting an emerging pathogen are low. Simply watch out for the usual germ hot spots at home, at work or school, and when out in social situations. For big events in your life, consider thinking about the potential for infection that might come about because of this change. No need to become a germophobe who obsesses over every perceived, however remote, chance of infection! Just make a quick assessment from time to time of the germ quotient in your life. Start this assessment by asking the following questions:

➤ Am I about to travel to a part of the world I have never visited before?

➤ Am I about to move to a new town or city more than two hundred miles from where I now live?

➤ Am I about to start a new job in this new city?

➤ Does my job now require increased air travel?

➤ Have I just moved into a new housing development or single home built on previously undisturbed land?

➤ Have I taken up a new hobby that puts me in an unfamiliar environment, such as gardening, mushroom collecting, scuba diving, spelunking, mountain climbing, horseback riding, or hunting?

➤ Have I just purchased a new pet?

➤ Has my community experienced a sudden increase in population?

The last question may lead to a controversial topic that you may find uncomfortable to discuss with others or even think about on your own. Does a connection exist between immigration and increased infection rates? From a strictly scientific viewpoint, the answer is yes. Remember, one of the reasons that diseases emerge in new populations relates to mass movements of people across the world. The combination of mass migrations and ignorance about germs can be deadly. These two factors keep many diseases alive that we should have long ago conquered, diseases such as STDs, TB, and even the flu.

Increasing Your Knowledge of Emerging Diseases

If you answered yes to any of the above questions, investigate the topic further. Do a little research on the types of germs you are likely to face by traveling to New Guinea, raising turtles, going on an archeological dig, or any other new activity you are about to tackle. With the Internet, there no longer exists any excuse for ignorance on almost any subject.

The following is hardly an exhaustive list, but it might give you an idea of where to begin learning about specific emerging diseases:

➤ International health agencies such as the WHO or the Pan American Health Organization

➤ National health agencies such as the CDC

➤ Local public health offices such as your state's or county's Department of Public Health

➤ Government offices such as the U.S. State Department

➤ Microbiology organizations such as the American Society for Microbiology or the Infectious Diseases Society of America

➤ Organizations or societies focused on specific hobbies, subjects, or activities, such as the Mycological Society of America, the American Kennel Club, or the American Veterinary Medical Association. These groups have contact information for experts who can answer specific germ-related questions.

Asking your family doctor should always be an option available to you if you are concerned about potential exposure to a new germ.

CHAPTER 24

Zoonotic Diseases— Diseases from Animals

In This Chapter

➤ How animals carry infectious disease

➤ Infections we get from our main animal reservoirs

➤ Getting to know your animal reservoirs

➤ The main pathogens of pets, farm animals, birds, and wildlife

➤ Tips for reducing your chance of getting a zoonotic disease

In this chapter you will become acquainted with the main zoonotic diseases that affect people in North America. If you were to travel the world, you would be exposed to animal populations that are different from those found on this continent. Thus, travelers should consider the types of zoonotic diseases prevalent at their destinations.

Zoonotic diseases comprise a very large topic within infectious disease. Animals play a major role as reservoirs of human diseases, including emerging diseases. Sometimes animals carry infectious agents straight into a human population, such as ground squirrels carrying the hantavirus. In other instances, an animal serves as the reservoir for the pathogen, which can be transmitted to people by another living thing. For example, the pathogen that causes bubonic plague stays in its rat reservoir until a flea bites the rat. The pathogen then moves into the flea, which can transmit it to humans with another bite.

People tend to forget that some infectious diseases go from humans to animals, too. For example, influenza moves back and forth between humans and pigs. People can also transmit several infections to primates, such as chimpanzees and monkeys.

Even if you do not own pets or livestock or plan on camping under the stars, you may know someone who does. Fighting infections is accomplished by blocking germ transmission, and that is much easier to do if you have a sense of where germs are lurking.

Animals that Carry Infectious Agents

Animals can be carriers of infection in exactly the same way people carry infectious agents. Thus, an animal can be an active, healthy (asymptomatic), convalescent, or incubatory carrier.

Animals carry these infectious agents either inside their bodies or on the outside on fur, hair, feathers, skin, or scales. For this reason, advice on fighting infections always includes washing hands after touching an animal or spending time at a place that houses animals (farms, zoos, petting zoos, etc.).

Animal-to-human transmission is usually by contact, vehicle, or airborne transmission, such as in the following examples:

> ➤ Contact transmission: Bites, scratches, licking, inhalation of droplets, and direct contact by touching live animals or hides, wool, pelts, or carcasses

> ➤ Vehicle transmission: Picking up pathogens from cages, pens, stalls, feeders, water buckets, grooming tools, or toys

> ➤ Airborne transmission: Breathing particles from feces or bioaerosols from sneezing or coughing

Animal Reservoirs

Almost any animal group you can imagine has the ability to carry an infectious agent, either by acting as a reservoir or by carrying the pathogen on the outside of its body. Animals have the potential to carry bacteria, viruses, fungi, protozoa, and parasites, and people who are at high risk for infection must be extra vigilant regarding animal germs, as they are with non-zoonotic pathogens.

The following animal groups carry at least one microbe that causes infection in humans:

➤ Amphibians

➤ Armadillos

➤ Bats

➤ Birds

➤ Cats

➤ Dogs

➤ Fish

➤ Hoofed animals

➤ Marine mammals

➤ Marsupials

➤ Nonhuman primates

➤ Rabbits

➤ Reptiles

➤ Rodents

➤ Swine

People who work with any of these animals receive professional advice on handling them and avoiding infection. Everyone else can avoid infection by staying away from many of these animals when there is any doubt about their health and care.

If you are not experienced in the care of any of these animals, it is a good idea to learn about the main zoonotic diseases that these animals carry.

Infections and Disease

Rabies is caused by the rabies virus. The disease is one of our most feared neurological disorders and rightly so because though rare, it is almost always fatal.

The main carriers of rabies are raccoons, skunks, bats, foxes, and coyotes. A bite from an infected animal can transmit the virus via the animal's saliva to humans. Inhalation of bat saliva droplets also leads to infection. Cattle, dogs, and cats that have been infected by being bitten by one of these animals can also transmit the virus to people. All of these domesticated animals (in most cases horses, too) should be vaccinated.

The symptoms of rabies vary among species. In dogs and other canines, cats, raccoons, and skunks, symptoms include the following:

➤ Abnormal nervousness

➤ Irritability

➤ Snapping

➤ Exaggerated response to noise or visual stimuli

Salivation increases as throat muscles become paralyzed. As the disease progresses, the animal will become disoriented, experience seizures, have trouble breathing, and emit a choking sound. Death usually comes because of respiratory failure due to muscle paralysis.

The incubation period varies widely depending on the species. In dogs, it can range from three weeks to six months. In cats, symptoms appear from two to six weeks. Humans experience a similar wide range in incubation period. Three to six weeks is an average incubation period in people, but it can last as long as a year after the initial infection.

Microbe Basics

The genus *Rickettsia* contains an unusual group of small bacteria (about 0.3 micrometer in width) that must infect other living cells to survive. When *Rickettsia* enters a host, it induces the phagocytes of the immune system to ingest it. Inside the phagocyte, *Rickettsia* is adept at avoiding the destructive enzymes associated with phagocytosis. The pathogens thus use phagocytes as a hiding place from other actions by the immune system.

Rickettsia reproduces slowly inside the cells it invades. By producing only about ten new offspring, the pathogen can prolong its time inside the host cell and stay under the immune system's radar. Although *Rickettsia* can invade any cell type, it prefers skin, brain, and heart tissue. The diseases collectively known as rickettsial diseases affect these tissues. They are caused mainly by species of the genera *Coxiella*, *Ehrlichia*, and *Bartonella*, in addition to *Rickettsia*.

Infections from Pets

Fido and Tabby may be your best friends, part of your family, and may even be named in your will. Try to remember that your cuddly friends also like to visit some fairly disgusting places in their free time. Anything that smells awful, looks like it might be dead, or wriggles, squeaks, squirms, or slithers holds endless fascination for them. Fido and Tabby also like to lick places that would best be left unlicked. They sometimes eat their wastes, or the wastes of others! After all these activities and explorations, they enjoy coming home to give you a big kiss.

We get infections from the most common furry pets (dogs, cats, guinea pigs, hamsters, rabbits, weasels, ferrets, rats, and mice) by contact with the animal or from an insect carried by the pet. People who keep birds, reptiles, and amphibians have a risk of infections that differ from those carried by furry animals, but the basic infection-fighting tips still apply.

All pet owners have a normal flora that reflects the pet that lives with them. Thus, if you own a dog, your normal flora probably has some dog microbes as part of its makeup. A cat owner has a slightly different composition that includes cat microbes, a stable owner has horse microbes, and so on. These comprise the beneficial flora that helps defend you against more serious infectious agents.

Let's start with the most common pets and the infection-causing microbes they might carry.

Microbe Basics

Puppies and adult dogs receive a standard regimen of vaccinations to protect their health and the health of their owners. The program may vary a bit depending on where you live. Mushers in Alaska have fewer worries about tropical diseases than pet owners in Florida. Beyond this common sense, ask your veterinarian's advice on the shots your dog should receive and their schedule. The required battery of vaccinations for dog diseases should be distemper, leptospirosis, parvovirus, and rabies. Many vets also add a vaccine for Lyme disease and kennel cough.

Many dog owners over-vaccinate Fido. Each vaccine has a schedule that works best for keeping your dog infection-free. For example, a rabies shot lasts for three years before needing a booster. Vaccinating your dog too frequently harms the dog and wastes your money.

Dog Germs

For dog owners, or any pet owner, always check with your veterinarian regarding the infections posing the greatest health risk or chance of transmission.

Infections or diseases can be carried by dogs and other canines, such as coyotes, wolves, or their hybrids. Following are the most common infections:

➤ Skin infections from *Staphylococcus* or *Streptococcus* bacterial infections at the site of a bite or scratch

➤ Sore throat from *Streptococcus pyogenes* infection

➤ Fever or rashes from *Rickettsia*, *Salmonella*, *Borrelia*, *Ehrlichia*, or *Leptospira* bacteria

➤ Diarrhea, general gastroenteritis, or a general illness with fever, chills, and diarrhea from *Campylobacter jejuni* or *Leptospira* bacteria

➤ Dermatitis (as tinea or ringworm) from fungi such as *Microsporum canis*

➤ Rabies caused by the rabies virus and transmitted by bites

Preventing bites is the best way to avoid serious infections from dogs. Follow these rules:

➤ Use caution around any unknown dog and do not take a threatening posture, such as prolonged direct eye contact, putting your face too close to the dog's face, or raising your arm as if to hit the animal

> ➤ Do not startle a sleeping dog or interfere with a dog when he is eating

> ➤ Do not leave children unattended with dogs

Although rabies from dogs is extremely rare because of good vaccination programs in the United States, the risk increases outside the United States. Avoid any dog showing signs of rabies. For your own dog, keep rabies vaccinations up to date and try to reduce any contact your dog has with wildlife or free-roaming dogs.

Cat Germs

Cats are the second most common house pet and have been human companions since the first recorded history, and likely earlier.

Cats carry some of the same pathogens as dogs. These common pathogens are the rabies virus, various tick-borne pathogens such as *Ehrlichia*, and *Salmonella* and *C. jejuni*. Following are the infections and diseases carried by cats that are of greatest concern:

> ➤ Cat scratch disease: A global disease of flulike symptoms caused by the bacterium *Bartonella*

> ➤ Toxoplasmosis: Caused by the protozoan *Toxoplasma gondii*, which is present as cysts in cat feces

> ➤ Q fever: A tick-borne disease caused by the bacterium *Coxiella burnetii*; cats tend to be asymptomatic

Microbe Basics

Kittens and adult cats need vaccinations based on their lifestyle. A cat that lives indoors requires a vaccination program different from one let loose all day on a farm or in your neighborhood.

Your veterinarian will decide on the best program for your cat based on the likelihood of exposure to infectious agents. The vaccines that might be recommended are rabies, feline panleukopenia virus, feline calicivirus, feline herpes virus, and feline leukemia virus. Your vet may also recommend vaccinating against ringworm and *Chlamydia* infections.

As with dogs, the feline rabies shot should last for three years before a booster is needed. The other vaccines follow their own specific schedules.

Exotic Pets

Exotic pets come from places far away and live as pets in situations very foreign to their normal climate, food, and predators and prey. If an exotic pet escapes from your care—or worse, if you release it intentionally—the pet will either soon die or will take over its surroundings, causing severe harm to native animals and plants. Escaped exotic pets also pose the risk of carrying infectious agents into native animal populations. As a result, exotic pets contribute to our loss of native species every year.

People hold different views on what constitutes an exotic pet. To some, weasels seem exotic, but another person may have raised them for years and knows much about weasel ways.

Before owning an exotic pet, seek information on the types of infections most likely to be carried by the animal. Ask a veterinarian about how to prevent infections in this animal and what to do in case you get infected.

The following are the pathogens associated with common exotic pets. This list is not exhaustive, so be sure to learn about the rarer diseases you could get from these pets:

➤ Amphibians and reptiles: Mainly salmonellosis, an infection from *Salmonella* bacteria; lizards also carry *Yersinia* bacteria

➤ Ferrets: Infections from *Salmonella* and *Campylobacter* bacteria, and influenza and SARS viral infections

➤ Gerbils: Mainly salmonellosis

➤ Guinea pigs: Bacterial infections from *Salmonella*, *Pasteurella*, and *Yersinia*; dermatophytosis from the fungus *Trichophyton*

➤ Hamsters: Bacterial infections from *Salmonella*, *Pasteurella*, and *Campylobacter*; various dermatophytoses

➤ Mice: Salmonellosis, dermatophytoses from the fungus *Trichophyton*, and infection from lymphocytic choriomeningitis (LCM) virus

➤ Rabbits: Infections from the bacteria *Pasteurella* and *Salmonella*, various dermatophytoses from the fungi *Trichophyton* and *Microsporum*, and viral infection from monkeypox

➤ Rats: Infections from *Pasteurella* and *Salmonella*, dermatophytosis from *Trichophyton*, and the viral infection hantavirus pulmonary syndrome

Owning nonhuman primates produces special health issues because pathogens go back and forth easily between humans and primates. The most common diseases that transmit between nonhuman primates and humans are the following:

- ➤ Hepatitis A and B
- ➤ Herpes
- ➤ Measles
- ➤ Salmonellosis
- ➤ Shigellosis
- ➤ Tuberculosis
- ➤ Various dermatophytoses caused by fungi
- ➤ Amoebiasis
- ➤ Balantidiasis

Microbe Basics

Tuberculosis (TB) is a severe infection of the lower respiratory tract. TB follows a long course in the body before a person returns to full health. A return to health can be assured only by taking a regimen of four drugs in a sequence prescribed by a doctor.

All TB is caused by *Mycobacterium*. This genus of bacteria contains about fifty known species, of which about thirty cause some form of disease. Because people are susceptible to more than one species that cause a similar type of disease, microbiologists group *Mycobacterium* into complexes:

- ➤ *M. tuberculosis* complex, consisting of *M. tuberculosis*, *M. aficanum*, *M. bovis*, and *M. microti*
- ➤ *M. leprae* complex, consisting of *M. leprae* and *M. lepromatosis*
- ➤ *M. avium* complex, consisting of *M. avium*, *M. intracellulare*, and *M. scrofulaceum*

The first two groups are most prevalent in humans. *M. tuberculosis* complex species cause TB and *M. leprae* complex species cause the disease leprosy.

Infections from Birds

Infections in birds can lead to disease in the bird and in humans. In many cases, the bird disease differs from the human disease. Influenza represents an important exception. The flu virus infects chickens, ducks, and various other waterfowl. In these birds, the flu is a respiratory disease as it is in humans, but it can also spread to the digestive tract and the nerves. In humans, the flu stays in the upper respiratory tract.

Owners of parrots and parakeets should become familiar with diseases transmitted from birds to humans. The following diseases affect birds and people:

➤ Psittacosis: Caused by *Chlamydia psittaci*, this is a respiratory and intestinal disease in birds and a respiratory illness in humans. It is transmitted by airborne movement of particles from dry feces.

➤ Newcastle disease: Caused by the Newcastle virus (related to the mumps virus), this affects the respiratory tract and nervous system in birds and causes conjunctivitis in people.

➤ Influenza: Bird flu affects several systems in the bird's body but only the respiratory tract in people. It is transmitted by airborne bioaerosols or droplets.

➤ Yersiniosis: Caused by the *Yersinia pseudotuberculosis* bacteria, this is an intestinal disease in both birds and people, transmitted in contaminated foods.

➤ West Nile disease: Caused by the West Nile virus carried by mosquitoes, this disease is fatal to many bird species, especially crows.

➤ Cryptococcosis: Caused by the yeast *Cryptococcus neoformans*; birds carry the pathogen in their intestines and usually do not get sick. It causes lower respiratory tract infection in people.

➤ Histoplasmosis: This emerging disease is caused by the fungus *Histoplasma capsulatum*. The natural source is soil, but the pathogen seems to be in higher levels in soils contaminated by bird droppings. People get histoplasmosis via airborne transmission of contaminated soil particles. This human disease resembles TB.

People who are exposed to domesticated birds should keep in mind that birds transmit pathogens in three ways:

➤ Airborne transmission of particles from feces

➤ Droplet contact transmission and inhalation of the pathogen

➤ Vector transmission by insects

Infections from Domesticated Farm Animals

Getting infections from farm animals is rare, but livestock can carry infectious agents so a little caution is recommended. Cattle carry a bacterium, *Mycobacterium bovis*, that is closely related to our TB microbe. Thus, exposure to cattle may slightly increase your risk of TB.

Manure contains a large amount of *E. coli*, including the virulent strain *E. coli* O157:H7. Cattle and calves are thought to be a major source of the *E. coli* O157:H7 that gets into our food and causes food-borne outbreaks. In fact, manure from farm animals also contains the food-borne pathogens *Campylobacter jejuni*, *Salmonella*, *Cryptosporidium*, and *Yersinia enterocolitica*.

You may also be at a higher risk of the following bacterial diseases that spread by airborne transmission or vector transmission from livestock to humans:

➤ Brucellosis caused by *Brucella*

➤ Q fever caused by *Coxiella burnetii*

➤ Leptospirosis caused by *Leptospira*

Another concern of hobnobbing with farm animals relates to anthrax. This disease is rare in the general population because most of us do not spend much time with livestock. But the chances of being exposed to this pathogen goes up if you spend time around cattle, horses, sheep, or other farm animals. The anthrax pathogen *Bacillus anthracis* lives in soil and not on animals, but livestock can get the microbe on their coat when they roll in contaminated pastures. This is true also for dogs and cats that live on a farm. Anthrax has a higher incidence in parts of the world where people live an agrarian lifestyle and are close to livestock daily.

The disease tetanus is caused by another soil microbe, *Clostridium tetani*, and has also been associated with farm life. Animals are not to blame for this one. Working on a farm usually leads to an assortment of cuts and scrapes. These breaks in your skin barrier open the door for *C. tetani* and its cousin *Clostridium perfringens*, which causes gangrene. Both of these bacteria are anaerobes, meaning they thrive in airless conditions. Wounds left untended and dirty contain numerous airless pockets where *Clostridium* can grow.

Any skin wound from activities on a farm or gardening, camping, hiking, or other outdoor activity should be cleaned immediately. Apply an antimicrobial cream if you have one. If not, consider pouring a few drops of alcohol-based hand sanitizer onto the wound to kill microbes. This will hurt for a few seconds, but the pain is less of a risk to you than tetanus or gangrene!

Infections from Wildlife

The main threat from wildlife is rabies. Any animal can carry this virus, so livestock and pets are not absolved, but you have a better chance of learning a domesticated animal's health history than that of wildlife.

The main health threat from wildlife after bites comes from insect-borne infections. Ticks, fleas, and mosquitoes carry many of humanity's worst infectious diseases. Veterinarians hold a wealth of knowledge on the types of infections most likely to reach you when you are exposed to wildlife. Wildlife, nonetheless, remains a great unknown in how infectious disease enters and leaves human populations.

Here are the better-known infections from wildlife:

> ➤ Rabies: Caused by the rabies virus and carried by various wildlife, especially small mammals

> ➤ Cryptosporidiosis: A severe diarrheal disease caused by *Cryptosporidium* cysts shed in animal feces and then contaminating surface waters

> ➤ Cryptococcosis: A respiratory infection caused by *C. neoformans* and *C. gattii* fungi. People get the pathogen by inhaling particles from dry bird droppings, especially from pigeons

> ➤ Plague: a fatal systemic disease caused by the bacterium *Yersinia pestis* and transmitted by fleas from its reservoir in rats to people

> ➤ Lyme disease: An infection causing flulike symptoms and transmitted from wildlife to people by ticks. Deer populations are known to be an important reservoir for the pathogen *Borrelia burgdorferi*

> ➤ Rocky Mountain spotted fever: Caused by the bacterium *Rickettsia rickettsii* and carried by ticks from various wildlife

> ➤ TB: Caused by various species of *Mycobacterium*. In addition to cattle, which carry *M. bovis*, TB species may be carried by elk, bison, and deer

Additional diseases confined to bird reservoirs are described in the above section on infections from birds.

Preventing zoonotic diseases may be one of the most difficult infection-fighting challenges you will face. Your chances of infection increase in proportion to your time spent with animals. The best first step in prevention is to know the health history of the animal. Pets and domesticated farm animals should receive an up-to-date program of vaccinations. If you are not sure if this has occurred, or if any animal behaves abnormally to suggest it is diseased, get away from the animal and call a veterinarian or an animal control office.

INDEX

H

N

The Smart Guide Series

Making Smart People Smarter

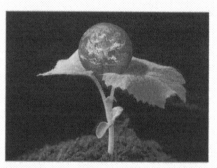

THE SMART GUIDE TO

GREEN LIVING

The most complete guide to green living ever published

How green living benefits your health as well as the Earth's

How green living can save you lots of money

Why the green economy and job market is an attractive, new, lucrative frontier

Julie Kerr **Gines**

Available Titles

Smart Guide To Astronomy
Smart Guide To Bachelorette Parties
Smart Guide To Back and Nerve Pain
Smart Guide To Biology
Smart Guide To Bridge
Smart Guide To Chemistry
Smart Guide To Classical Music
Smart Guide To Deciphering A Wine Label
Smart Guide To eBay
Smart Guide To Fighting Infections
Smart Guide To Forensic Careers
Smart Guide To Forensic Science
Smart Guide To Freshwater Fishing
Smart Guide To Getting Published
Smart Guide To Golf
Smart Guide To Green Living
Smart Guide To Healthy Grilling
Smart Guide To High School Math
Smart Guide To Hiking and Backpacking
Smart Guide To Horses and Riding
Smart Guide To Life After Divorce
Smart Guide To Making A Fortune With Infomercials
Smart Guide To Managing Stress
Smart Guide To Medical Imaging Tests
Smart Guide To Nutrition
Smart Guide To Patents
Smart Guide To Practical Math
Smart Guide To Single Malt Scotch
Smart Guide To Starting Your Own Business
Smart Guide To The Perfect Job Interview
Smart Guide To The Solar System
Smart Guide To Understanding Your Cat
Smart Guide To US Visas
Smart Guide To Wedding Weekend Events
Smart Guide To Wine

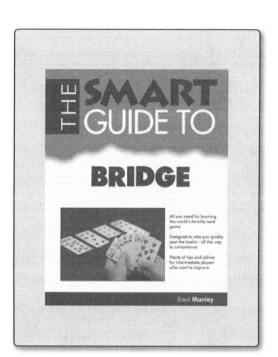

THE SMART GUIDE TO

BRIDGE

All you need for learning
the world's favorite card
game

Designed to take you quickly
past the basics – all the way
to competence

Plenty of tips and advice
for intermediate players
who want to improve

Brent Manley

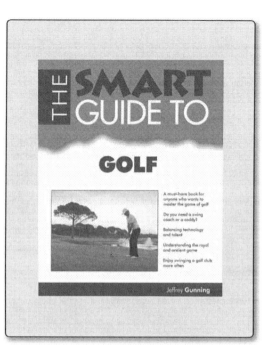

THE SMART GUIDE TO

GOLF

A must-have book for
anyone who wants to
master the game of golf

Do you need a swing
coach or a caddy?

Balancing technology
and talent

Understanding the royal
and ancient game

Enjoy swinging a golf club
more often

Jeffrey Gunning

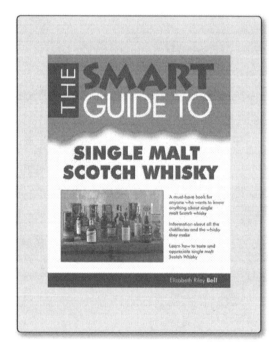

THE SMART GUIDE TO

SINGLE MALT
SCOTCH WHISKY

A must-have book for
anyone who wants to know
anything about single
malt Scotch whisky

Information about all the
distilleries and the whisky
they make

Learn how to taste and
appreciate single malt
Scotch Whisky

Elizabeth Riley Bell

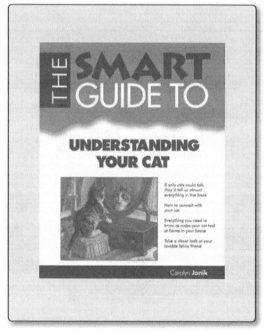

THE SMART GUIDE TO

UNDERSTANDING
YOUR CAT

If only cats could talk,
they'd tell us almost
everything in this book

How to connect with
your cat

Everything you need to
know to make your cat feel
at home in your home

Take a closer look at your
lovable feline friend

Carolyn Janik

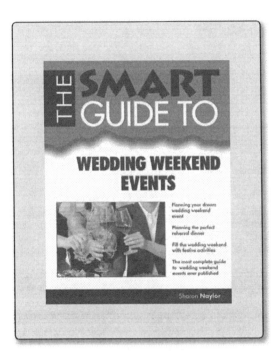

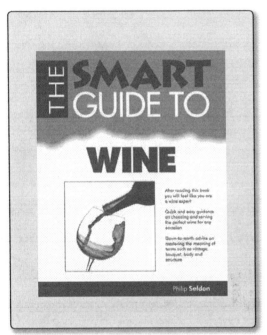

The Smart Guide Series

Making Smart People Smarter

Smart Guides are available at your local bookseller

or from the following Internet retailers

www.SmartGuidePublications.com

www.Amazon.com

www.BarnesandNoble.com

Smart Guides are popularly priced from $18.95

Smart Guides are also available in Kindle and Nook editions

ABOUT THE AUTHOR

Anne Maczulak

Author of The Smart Guide To Fighting Infections, The Smart Guide To Nutrition, and The Smart Guide to Biology

Anne Maczulak, PhD, is the author of over 10 books on biology and ecology including Allies and Enemies: How the World Depends on Bacteria, and The Five-Second Rule and Other Myths about Germs. Anne has contributed to articles on germophobia, the fear of germs, in *Psychology Today* and has been a regular guest on television and radio, speaking to viewers about the good and bad microbes that lurk in households. As a regular guest expert on Martha Stewart Living Radio (Sirius/XM Radio), Anne answers callers' questions on disinfectants, infection, food-borne germs, and other topics in germ-fighting. Anne has spoken to professional hygiene organizations on the best ways to disinfect surfaces. She consults for drug and biotechnology companies as well as laboratories that test new antimicrobial products.

Anne's audiences benefit from her ability to transform complex subjects into easy-to-understand lessons. And yet, reading Anne's books on biology, ecology, and microbiology never feels like reading a textbook. Anne always relates technical topics to the "big picture" and writes for non-scientists.

Anne's talent in making connections between seemingly unrelated topics in biology comes from her background in nutrition and microbiology. As a PhD in nutrition with a specialty in microbiology, Anne studied the relationship between intestinal microbes and how humans and other animals use nutrients. During her career in industry, Anne studied microbes of the skin and scalp, the bacteria in drinking water, and microbes of the environment that produce useful cold-tolerant enzymes.

Visit her website www.AnneMaczulak.com for more on her books and to keep up on "News for Germophiles" and "News for Germophobes."

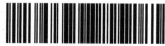

Made in the USA
Charleston, SC
27 May 2012